O P L

OXFORD PSYCHIATRY LIBRARY

C000066336

Sports Psychiatry

O P L

OXFORD PSYCHIATRY LIBRARY

Sports Psychiatry

Edited by

Dr Alan Currie

Consultant Psychiatrist, Northumberland Tyne and
Wear NHS Foundation Trust, St Nicholas Hospital, Gosforth,
Newcastle upon Tyne, UK;
Honorary Clinical Lecturer, Newcastle University,
Newcastle upon Tyne, UK

Dr Bruce Owen

Consultant Psychiatrist and Director of Medical Education,
Northumberland Tyne and Wear NHS Foundation Trust,
St Nicholas Hospital, Gosforth, Newcastle upon Tyne, UK;
Honorary Clinical Lecturer, Newcastle University,
Newcastle upon Tyne, UK

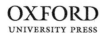

OXFORD
UNIVERSITY PRESS

Great Clarendon Street, Oxford, OX2 6DP,
United Kingdom

Oxford University Press is a department of the University of Oxford.
It furthers the University's objective of excellence in research, scholarship,
and education by publishing worldwide. Oxford is a registered trade mark of
Oxford University Press in the UK and in certain other countries

© Oxford University Press 2016

The moral rights of the authors have been asserted

Impression: 1

All rights reserved. No part of this publication may be reproduced, stored in
a retrieval system, or transmitted, in any form or by any means, without the
prior permission in writing of Oxford University Press, or as expressly permitted
by law, by licence or under terms agreed with the appropriate reprographics
rights organization. Enquiries concerning reproduction outside the scope of the
above should be sent to the Rights Department, Oxford University Press, at the
address above

You must not circulate this work in any other form
and you must impose this same condition on any acquirer

Published in the United States of America by Oxford University Press
198 Madison Avenue, New York, NY 10016, United States of America

British Library Cataloguing in Publication Data

Data available

Library of Congress Control Number: 2015947234

ISBN 978–0–19–873462–8

Printed in Great Britain by
Clays Ltd, St Ives plc

Oxford University Press makes no representation, express or implied, that the
drug dosages in this book are correct. Readers must therefore always check
the product information and clinical procedures with the most up-to-date
published product information and data sheets provided by the manufacturers
and the most recent codes of conduct and safety regulations. The authors and
the publishers do not accept responsibility or legal liability for any errors in the
text or for the misuse or misapplication of material in this work. Except where
otherwise stated, drug dosages and recommendations are for the non-pregnant
adult who is not breast-feeding

Links to third party websites are provided by Oxford in good faith and
for information only. Oxford disclaims any responsibility for the materials
contained in any third party website referenced in this work.

Foreword

The field of sports psychiatry has been developing steadily in recent years and we are now seeing the emergence of a specialist discipline that requires specific knowledge, skills, and approaches. As elite and grass-roots sports are calling upon psychiatrists to provide a service to their athletes and staff, there is a need to consolidate current psychiatric understanding and offer guidance from shared experience in the field.

This is the first comprehensive sports psychiatry handbook and it will be an invaluable practical guide for many. What Dr Currie and Dr Owen have done within this volume of work is to draw together current knowledge that will direct the efforts of a range of practitioners for the benefit of the health and performance of athletes. This book will be of immense value not only to psychiatrists but also to the many other experts working within sport, such as sports specialist doctors, psychologists, specialist sports psychologists, physiotherapists, strength and conditioning coaches, nutritionists, performance directors, coaches, team leaders, and athletes alike. The book will also allow professionals who work outside of sport to understand the particular difficulties that can be encountered in the sporting arena and some of the solutions to these.

The breadth of topics covered includes insights and practical ways of managing the spectrum of anxiety states and mood disorders that are so often seen in the sporting context. There are very helpful chapters covering eating disorders, addictions and addictive behaviours, alongside the more recently emphasized adult attention deficit hyperactivity disorder presentations, and a chapter exploring the impact of an athlete's personality on their health and performance. Later chapters address the sporting arena and the benefits of sport in general, and the book concludes with a review of drug prescribing within sport.

As a psychiatrist who has spent considerable time working in elite sport I can say that this book is a very welcome addition to my own collection. I strongly recommend it to colleagues working within the sporting field and anyone who has an interface with sport and with athletes. It will lead the emerging field of sports psychiatry and is a landmark in driving forward the importance of good mental health in sport, as in life.

Professor Steve Peters

Preface

We believe that sport is important. It is good for individuals and for their mental and physical well-being. It is good for personal development, for learning lessons, and for developing resilience; all of which are transferable to other areas of life. It is good for friendships and relationships. It is good for communities and it is good for societies.

We are equally aware that providing good mental health care can be challenging at the best of times and that these challenges are no less present in a sporting environment. Even if expertise is readily available there may still be individual, organizational, and practical obstacles to accessing this. We wish to equip all the health professionals who work in sport with a sufficient understanding of how mental illness can present and how it can be managed to ensure that the mental health needs of athletes are met in the same manner as their other health needs.

It is unusual for a sports club or team or even for a national governing body to have its own psychiatrist (although this is becoming more common). When a patient sees a psychiatrist it is important that the psychiatrist assesses not only the illness but also the individual and the context in which the condition has arisen and developed. These are basic competencies in any health professional. When the patient is an athlete, sport will form a large part of that context and an understanding of sport will be critical to a full and helpful formulation of the presenting problem. We hope we have addressed mental health problems in sport to a sufficient degree that this will be possible for all psychiatrists and that no athlete will feel compelled to say 'My psychiatrist doesn't understand me'.

It is common in many healthcare systems for psychiatrists to concentrate their time and clinical endeavours on those most disabled and marginalized by mental illness. It is here that sport can be harnessed as the route to recovery and to a more inclusive life. For this to succeed, the role of sport and of sports organizations has to be understood and appreciated by mental health specialists.

We believe that mental health is important. We want the range of professionals working in sport to have the knowledge and expertise necessary to address the needs of athletes. We want mental health professionals to be able to help athletes when called and to know how to promote sport as a route to better mental health.

It has been a privilege to collaborate with the many experts who have contributed to the chapters in this book and we have appreciated their wisdom and guidance. We hope it is valuable to you wherever you work and whatever your professional background.

Alan Currie and Bruce Owen

Contents

vii

Contents

Abbreviations

ADHD	attention deficit hyperactivity disorder
BAP	British Association for Psychopharmacology
BMD	bone mineral density
BMI	body mass index
CBT	cognitive behavioural therapy
DSM-5	Diagnostic and Statistical Manual of Mental Disorders, fifth edition
EA	energy availability
EI	energy intake
EPO	erythropoietin
FFM	fat-free mass
HPA	hypothalamic–pituitary–adrenal
HPG	hypothalamic–pituitary–gonadal
ICD-10	International Classification of Diseases, 10th revision
IPS	ideal performance state
IPT	interpersonal psychotherapy
MDD	major depressive disorder
NICE	National Institute for Health and Care Excellence
OCD	obsessive–compulsive disorder
OR	over-reaching
OTS	overtraining syndrome
PED	performance-enhancing drug
RED-S	relative energy deficiency in sport
SNRI	serotonin–noradrenaline reuptake inhibitor
SSRI	selective serotonin reuptake inhibitor
TUE	Therapeutic Use Exemption
WADA	World Anti-Doping Agency

Contributors

Jon Arcelus

Consultant Psychiatrist and Honorary Professor in Psychiatry, Division of Psychiatry and Applied Psychology, Faculty of Medicine & Health Sciences, Institute of Mental Health, University of Nottingham, Nottingham, UK and Nottingham National Centre for Gender Dysphoria, Nottingham, UK

Sarah Broadhead

Chartered Psychologist, Director of Sport, Chimp Management Ltd, Chapel en le Frith, Derbyshire, UK

Alan Currie

Consultant Psychiatrist, Northumberland Tyne and Wear NHS Foundation Trust, St Nicholas Hospital, Gosforth, Newcastle upon Tyne, UK and Honorary Clinical Lecturer, Newcastle University, Newcastle upon Tyne, UK

Kate Goodger

Chartered Psychologist, Director of Education, Chimp Management Ltd, Chapel en le Frith, UK

Andrea Hearn

Consultant Psychiatrist, Northumberland Tyne and Wear NHS Foundation Trust, St Nicholas Hospital, Gosforth, Newcastle upon Tyne, UK

Allan Johnston

Consultant Psychiatrist, Derbyshire Healthcare NHS Foundation Trust, Chesterfield, UK

Reshad Malik

Academic Clinical Fellow in Psychiatry, Camden and Islington NHS Foundation Trust, London, UK

Valentin Z. Markser

Psychiatrist, Psychotherapist, and Psychoanalyst, Institute for Sport Psychiatry, Cologne, Germany

R. Hamish McAllister-Williams

Reader in Clinical Psychopharmacology and Honorary Consultant Psychiatrist, Newcastle University, Newcastle upon Tyne, UK

Paul McArdle

Consultant Psychiatrist, Northumberland Tyne and Wear NHS Foundation Trust, St Nicholas Hospital, Gosforth, Newcastle upon Tyne, UK

David R. McDuff

Clinical Professor of Psychiatry, University of Maryland School of Medicine, Baltimore, MD, USA

Bruce Owen

Consultant Psychiatrist and Director of Medical Education, Northumberland Tyne and Wear NHS Foundation Trust, St Nicholas Hospital, Gosforth, Newcastle upon Tyne, UK and Honorary Clinical Lecturer, Newcastle University, Newcastle upon Tyne, UK

Carolyn Plateau

Lecturer in Psychology, School of Sport, Exercise and Health Sciences, Loughborough University, Loughborough, UK

Pamela Walters

Consultant in Forensic and Addiction Psychiatry, South London & Maudsley NHS Foundation Trust, London, & South West London & St Georges Mental Health NHS Trust, UK

Chapter 1

Adjustment and anxiety disorders

David R. McDuff

Key points

- A degree of anxiety is a normal and necessary part of training and competition. Some athletes develop more pervasive symptoms and may have an anxiety disorder needing comprehensive evaluation.
- Anxiety disorders are the most common mental disorders seen in sport and occur in two distinct groups—adjustment anxiety and primary anxiety disorders.
- Important co-morbid conditions such as depressive disorders, substance misuse, and attention deficit hyperactivity disorder may be present.
- Adjustment anxiety develops in relation to an identifiable stressor and usually last for weeks to months. Primary anxiety disorders are more chronic.
- Adjustment anxiety disorders are commonly seen as one of four subtypes with prominent symptoms of insomnia, depression, aggression, or somatization.
- Primary anxiety disorders include specific phobias, social anxiety, generalized anxiety, panic disorder, and obsessive–compulsive disorder.
- The recommended treatment approach is a collaborative model between the psychiatrist, medical team, and support staff (including the coach).
- Brief or time-limited therapies such as behavioural, cognitive behavioural, and/or motivational enhancement augmented by medication work best.
- If the natural social support groups around an athlete are utilized and symptoms are identified early, then outcomes are excellent.

1.1 Introduction

Anxiety typically manifests itself in three areas:

1. Cognitive anxiety—results in overanalysing; negative, doubtful, or comparative thinking; and preoccupation with mistakes, losses, or failure.
2. Disrupted focus and concentration—leads to diminished visual acuity, increased distractibility, and attention shifting that is slowed and erratic.
3. Somatic anxiety—results from physiological arousal and includes symptoms of rapid breathing and heart rate; light-headedness or dizziness; muscle tightness,

tremor, and altered movement mechanics; indigestion, abdominal discomfort, or diarrhoea; excess sweating; numbness or tingling; and excessive focus on pain or stiffness in an injured area.

In most competitors, symptoms are mild, manageable, and occur just before or in the first moments of predictably high-pressure situations (see Chapter 2). For others, however, anxiety occurs at higher levels throughout important practices, trials, or competitions and extends into other social, educational, or high-pressure activities. Symptoms tend to worsen when the athlete moves to a higher competitive level or enters periods of sustained stress, for example, in response to other life events or adjustments. When anxiety is disruptive to functioning in and out of sports and persists over weeks or months or longer, then one of the two main types of anxiety disorder (the adjustment type and the primary type) should be considered and a formal evaluation completed.

Adjustment anxiety disorders are common and clearly tied to significant stressors such as demotion, performance slump, injury, illness, loss, break-up/divorce, or financial distress. Anxiety is commonly accompanied by symptoms such as insomnia, depression, aggression, and somatization and sometimes triggered or aggravated by substance misuse (e.g. alcohol, stimulants, or cannabis).

Primary anxiety disorders are variable in presentation and can arise in childhood, adolescence, or adulthood and can be triggered or aggravated by sports participation. The most common ones seen in sports are specific phobias, social/performance anxiety, generalized anxiety, and panic. Obsessive–compulsive disorder (OCD) is usually classified along with the anxiety disorders. In its full clinical form there is severe functional impairment but it is less often encountered in sporting populations.

Each of these specific primary anxiety disorders can be aggravated by other medical problems or by the misuse of substances, especially stimulants or sedative hypnotics.

1.2 **Adjustment anxiety subtypes**

These are more common than primary anxiety disorders and tend to be seen as one of four subtypes (see Figure 1.1):

- Anxiety accompanied by insomnia—often the result of an overactive mind and pessimistic/fatalistic perspective.

- Anxiety with aggression—often associated with a volatile relationship with infidelity. Substance intoxication with alcohol, cannabis, or stimulants may be a factor.

- Anxiety with depression—here there is typically a prolonged period of poor performance or a demotion or significant loss.

- Anxiety and somatization (e.g. excessive pain, preoccupation with an injured area, or hesitancy during rehabilitation) is usually seen following a serious injury or re-injury or with a chronic condition that limits participation. Often the anxiety and somatic concerns fluctuate in intensity with the athlete's overall stress level.

They occur in 15–20% of athletes per year and most can be identified and treated if appropriate mental health expertise is easily available and integrated into the team's medical services.

Each subtype typically has one or more clear stressors and they are sometimes induced or aggravated by substance misuse. The focus of treatment is on managing

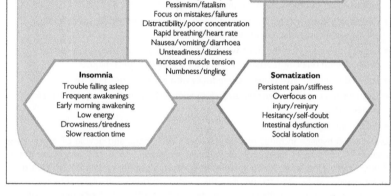

Aggression
Reactive anger
Fear of losing control
Sensitivity to criticism
Restless/muscle aches
Sense of unfairness
Blaming others
Heavy substances

Depression
Sadness/disappointment
Low energy/motivation
Poor concentration
Thoughts about
failure/death/suicide
Low self-esteem
Self-criticism

Adjustment anxiety
Overthinking/worrying
Pessimism/fatalism
Focus on mistakes/failures
Distractibility/poor concentration
Rapid breathing/heart rate
Nausea/vomiting/diarrhoea
Unsteadiness/dizziness
Increased muscle tension
Numbness/tingling

Insomnia
Trouble falling asleep
Frequent awakenings
Early morning awakening
Low energy
Drowsiness/tiredness
Slow reaction time

Somatization
Persistent pain/stiffness
Overfocus on
injury/reinjury
Hesitancy/self-doubt
Intestinal dysfunction
Social isolation

Figure 1.1 Adjustment anxiety subtypes.

the stressors, social support, supportive or motivational psychotherapy, and reducing symptoms and substance misuse through behavioural strategies and medication.

1.2.1 Assessment

Assessment involves a detailed history of current and past stressors, current stress symptoms, and attempts at stress control. A structured approach is recommended including symptom screening that asks about anxiety, depression, sleep, anger, mood, eating, pain, attention, and substance misuse. If any symptom area is positive then a formal rating scale can be useful (Beck Anxiety or Depression Inventories, the Epworth Sleepiness Scale, and/or the Campbell Domestic Violence Danger Assessment).

In addition, background information should be obtained:

- Support networks
- Personality style (e.g. perfectionism, obsessive/compulsive traits, distrust, social avoidance, low self-esteem, and emotional reactivity)
- Prior traumatic events and losses
- Family and cultural background
- Patterns of alcohol, caffeine, nicotine, cannabis, sedative or sleeping pills (over the counter and prescribed), and stimulants (prescribed (e.g. modafinil, methylphenidate, or amphetamines) or illicit (e.g. cocaine or methamphetamine)).

1.2.2 **Anxiety and insomnia**

This subtype usually occurs in an active thinker and worrier who doesn't have good problem-solving skills and/or an adequate support network. Typical stressors include concerns about making the team, conflicts with family members or partners, concern about an injury, and/or parenting a newborn. The most common symptoms are an overactive mind, distractibility, poor concentration, fear of a bad outcome, muscle tension, and difficulty switching off at night.

Interventions aim to turn off active thinking and worrying to allow restful sleep. Behavioural strategies include instruction about the following:

- Relaxation breathing (in through the nose four, hold seven, and out through the mouth eight; smoothly for eight-breath cycles)

- Resetting breathing (nasal hyperventilation—three 20-second sets with a long exhalation through the mouth after each)

- Gravity stretching (on the floor with arms and legs outstretched and externally rotated) with relaxation breathing—in four, out eight—for 3 minutes

- Full body dynamic stretching like windmills with good clearing breaths

- Strategic mini static or dynamic stretch breaks while seated with eyes closed for 60 seconds

- A 20-minute power nap.

Good sleep hygiene includes making the room dark, cool, and devoid of aggravating sounds. Avoid eating, exercising, or watching excessive TV/videos or gaming in the 2 hours before bedtime. Pleasing white noise from a cell phone application or a bedside machine can be used to stimulate the auditory circuitry and inhibit active thinking. Substances like alcohol, caffeine, and nicotine that are known to block sleep must also be reduced or eliminated. Bedtime should also be at the same time throughout the week and no later than midnight if possible.

Medication may be helpful although it is usually only considered alongside psychological treatments. The options include a trial of a selective serotonin reuptake inhibitor (SSRI) as a medium- to long-term treatment which is reserved for cases where psychological and short-term measures have been only partially effective. These drugs have a delayed onset of action of some weeks but are an effective, evidence-based treatment. More rapidly acting drugs include low-dose benzodiazepines such as diazepam or alprazolam which may be helpful but have addictive potential and should only be used in the short term. Sleep medication can be used alone or as an adjunct to benzodiazepines. These include zopiclone 7.5 mg when necessary (prn) 30 to 45 minutes before bedtime or trazodone 25, 50, or 75 mg prn 60–90 minutes prior to bedtime and 3–5 days a week.

1.2.3 **Anxiety and aggression**

This subtype may be found alongside a past history of reactive anger, sensitivity to criticism or rejection, disinhibition from heavy drinking, or irritability from stimulant/cannabis use. Typical stressors include an arrest, fighting or jealousy in a key relationship, financial mismanagement, intense competition for a place on a team, or participation in important end-of-season competitions. Common symptoms are negative thinking, a sense of unfairness, worrying, arousal (especially muscle tension), restlessness, irritability, and a fear of losing control or of a bad outcome. A specific assessment for potential domestic violence should be conducted if the athlete is in a relationship or with children. Impulsive anger is not exclusive to male athletes and is seen in women too. A screening tool for risk factors for partner violence can be used (the Campbell Domestic Violence Danger Assessment).

Behavioural strategies for this subtype target the management of existing stressors and the worry–stressed–angry–hurt–acting out vicious cycles that are typical. Stressors such as conflict in a relationship or parenting strain may need couples therapy or involvement of family members/friends for additional support.

When there are financial difficulties, consultation with a financial advisor or parents is needed. There may be poor money management with excessive spending on partying or gambling, financial support provided unwisely to extended family and friends, and child support.

Careful inquiry into the role that substances like alcohol, stimulants (prescribed or illicit), and cannabis use might play is important. If a substance use disorder or a behavioural addiction (e.g. gambling, gaming, or compulsive sexual promiscuity) is identified, then the involvement of an addiction specialist is often warranted.

When sustained poor athletic performance and/or conflicts with coaches are present, these are often perceived as threats to self-image and need to be addressed. Consultation with the coach (with the permission of the player) is advisable. A plan for improving performance, including mental training and conflict resolution, can be developed.

For recurring cycles of worrying and reactive anger, prompt action that integrates behavioural therapy, medication, and the athlete's support network is the recommended approach. Cognitive behavioural techniques can be helpful to increase self-awareness of rising worry, frustration, and stress. With practice, simple measures can be effective. The athlete can learn to insert a word phrase in a lowered voice like 'chill out' or 'easy' along with a behavioural break like changing the subject, walking away, or calling a friend. If these approaches are not effective, the involvement of a professional with specific expertise in anger management is advised.

It goes without saying that when there is a serious risk of domestic violence, weapons like firearms and knives must be removed and reduction or avoidance of intoxicants must be ensured.

Some medications are useful adjuncts to behavioural and supportive approaches. Ready access to a psychiatrist makes it easier to manage medication and integrate this with other therapy and support:

- Worrying and aggression—low-dose SSRIs like sertraline or escitalopram along with buspirone as needed
- Anger decompression—an antihistamine such as hydroxyzine or diphenhydramine
- Reactive anger reduction—regular gabapentin or lamotrigine
- Insomnia—trazodone
- Alcohol cravings—naltrexone, disulfiram, or acamprosate (see Chapter 5).

1.2.4 Anxiety and depression

This subtype usually occurs in a person who is sensitive to criticism and has chronic low self-esteem. They tend to isolate themselves when stressed and don't seek help until symptoms are more severe. There can often be a trigger, particularly a loss event. If so, the athlete can find it helpful to describe the importance and meaning of the loss and discuss where they are in the grieving process. If there has been a demotion, loss of contract, or non-selection then the relationship of this to self-esteem, confidence, and short- and long-term goals should be discussed.

Typical symptoms are constant worrying, arousal, insomnia, sadness, disappointment, crying, poor concentration, low energy and motivation, social isolation, thoughts of dying or escape, and attempted self-injury. Poor sleep patterns with low energy and tobacco, alcohol, or cannabis use can trigger significant symptom worsening over days or weeks.

It is important to address worrying and insomnia as these symptoms drive most others. As improvement occurs, perspective develops and the event can be seen a temporary adversity, perhaps with potential for personal growth and maturity.

For symptoms of excessive worrying, grounding techniques (e.g. meditation, yoga, or lying supine on the floor with legs and arms outstretched) and positive self-talk are all helpful. Athletes can be taught that if they turn on automatic functions like breathing, stretching, watching, or listening, then worrying can be inhibited. The athlete can be taught progressive muscle relaxation or stretching with synchronized breathing, distraction through exercise, music, books on tape, or short naps. Socialization (forced if necessary) with family, teammates, or friends is often helpful as is involvement of a family member or teammate in the treatment process as a motivator of change and monitor of progress.

For positive self-talk it is important to identify short phrases that activate positive emotions and hope (e.g. 'I can handle this', 'Ask for help, I have support', 'This pain will pass and I will learn important lessons', and 'A good night's sleep makes every tough situation better').

When substance misuse is evident this can be addressed using motivational strategies to develop the idea that despite temporary relief, substance misuse becomes part of the problem over time and a barrier to improvement.

For insomnia, techniques as described in Section 1.2.2 are again helpful. Handouts on stress control, sleep tips, and the effects of substances can be useful. A good unwinding routine that lasts about 60–90 minutes is critical for sleep during high-stress periods. Key components include low lighting, reduced stimulation (e.g. from mobile phones and computers), short rest or stretch, easy activities (reading, listening to music, writing a letter or in a journal), watching interesting or calming TV, and cooling the room down.

If behavioural strategies are helpful but improvement is insufficient, then medication should be added. First-line medication would be a trial of antidepressant treatment, with an SSRI although a serotonin–noradrenaline reuptake inhibitor (SNRI) can also be useful. These should be given for at least 3–6 months. Low-dose benzodiazepines can offer short-term relaxation but their addictive potential limits their use. Antihistamines are usually avoided since they may cause sedation and reduce reaction time. For insomnia, low-dose hypnotics can be tried, again as a short-term measure.

1.2.5 Anxiety and somatization

This subtype usually occurs in a person who internalizes emotions and typically experiences stress in an organ or an organ system. The most common somatic symptoms are:

- myofascial pain (e.g. tension headaches, neck and back tightness)

- intestinal dysfunction with pain, bloating, or diarrhoea
- neurological symptoms like dizziness, weakness, or numbness
- prolonged injury recovery with self-reported pain that is out of proportion to the injury or objective findings on examination.

Typical stressors are re-injury, loss of playing time, conflicts with family or coaches, or transition out of competition. Common symptoms are worrying about the future, fear of re-injury, insomnia, fatigue, muscle tension, dizziness, blaming others, social isolation, and persistent pain. These individuals continually scan their bodies for signals of distress and are able to focus strongly on one or more anatomical areas. They are often hypersensitive to touch when examined. A thorough discussion of the history of the injury and its treatment and questions about the athlete's expectations of the healing process and return to play is necessary. If an injury is not present then a complete stress history as described earlier should be taken with a special focus on possible conflicts with coaches or teammates and off-the-field worries.

It is important to validate the athlete's somatic concerns and ensure an adequate evaluation by an experienced sports medicine physician. Sometimes it is helpful to have an additional opinion from, for example, a sports chiropractor or physiotherapist for a different perspective and approach—although in practice the athlete may already have sought multiple opinions.

Old records including imaging studies should be obtained and reviewed in the athlete's presence. Misconceptions and misunderstandings are common and so it is important to discuss their understanding of the injury, its treatments, and prognosis and to cross-check this with the treating physician.

Symptoms should be monitored prospectively using a symptom tracker (a simple table or monthly calendar) with daily severity ratings, stress levels, and sleep quality. This allows the association between pain levels and high stress or poor sleep to be clearly established.

If chronic pain is the problem, many do not appreciate that there may be a significant myofascial component that will respond to stretching, icing/heating, active release techniques, ultrasound, or electrical stimulation.

For other symptoms like chest tightness, dizziness, or gastrointestinal activation then it can be helpful to try a hyperventilation provocation test (30–60 seconds of deep and rapid mouth–mouth breathing with strong inspiration) to reproduce symptoms followed by relaxation breathing (long clearing breaths) to eliminate them.

Short-term (3–6 months and 10–20 sessions) supportive therapy and work on stress control is often helpful to reduce symptoms, manage stressors, and identify solutions. If substance misuse is also present then this must be addressed.

Medications and other somatic strategies like therapeutic massage, acupuncture, and portable electrical stimulation can be included initially or later. Pain must be managed and regular use of a non-steroidal anti-inflammatory drug in combination with the physiotherapy is often effective. It is sometimes necessary to use a short course of steroids, muscle relaxants, or opioid pain medication (used in combination with a muscle relaxant in the evening for unwinding). These regimens can often break up a chronic cycle of post-injury pain.

If gastrointestinal activation symptoms are present then an agent that slows gastrointestinal motility like dicycloverine (dicyclomine—an antimuscarinic antispasmodic) or trazodone can be helpful.

Case study 1

A 35-year-old professional tennis player had her previous season ended by a serious ankle injury. She was worried that her coach had given up on her. She was so preoccupied with this that she was making more mistakes in practice and in games. She was not sleeping well and was lacking energy towards the end of practice.

Assessment: a thorough history of her ankle injury revealed that it was due to overtraining. Prior to practice (which typically lasted 2 hours), she would have an intense, repetitive 90-minute workout supervised by another trainer. She was so busy that she often skipped breakfast and would grab only a light snack prior to her afternoon practice. She would try to boost her energy by drinking large cups of coffee (400 mg of caffeine each) before workouts and after practice. Furthermore, she did not adequately resupply her fluids, electrolytes, or carbohydrates after practice. At home she was constantly worried about her lack of success and her coach's apparent loss of interest, and couldn't sleep. She tried to quieten her mind by watching television or using the Internet and would have two or three glasses of wine to unwind. A few hours after falling asleep, she would wake up feeling frustrated.

Intervention: her daily workout routines were reduced to three times a week and she structured in a recovery day. She found a sports physiotherapist and developed a comprehensive rehabilitation programme for her ankle. Her nutritional pattern was restructured with breakfast, lunch, and recovery drinks/snacks after workouts and practice. Her caffeine use was reduced to one or two smaller cups of coffee a day (400 mg total caffeine versus 1200 mg) and a more extensive unwinding routine was developed that reduced her TV/computer time and replaced it with reading, music, and stretching. She was seen every other week for ten sessions to focus on stress control and life balance. Since her worrying seemed so intense and had been present at moderate levels for several years, a trial of venlafaxine tapering up to 112.5 mg daily was initiated.

Her worrying and anxiety reduced, her sleep pattern improved, and she felt happier. She began to socialize more. As her anxiety diminished, the focus shifted to mental training in relaxation, focus and attention, visualization, positive self-talk, maintaining composure, intensity regulation, and goal setting. She learned these quickly and began to apply them both to her tennis and more generally in her life.

1.3 Primary anxiety disorders

The primary anxiety disorders can develop at any age but commonly appear at subclinical or mild levels in adolescence and young adulthood before coming to clinical attention later. In sports, these may start out as performance concerns and over time generalize to other life areas or they may be generalized from the outset. Primary anxiety disorders may co-occur with attention deficit hyperactivity disorder (ADHD) and with depressive disorders.

1.3.1 Specific phobias

There is often a background of separation anxiety or childhood phobias (e.g. fear of darkness, storms, dogs, or insects). Phobic anxiety is commonly seen in athletes on teams that travel extensively by plane and is often triggered by a problem on a flight. Fear of re-injury can also develop following a severe injury (e.g. complicated concussion, catastrophic collision requiring surgery, or prolonged rehabilitation with pain) and is accompanied by hesitancy, overthinking, and self-doubt.

Assessment consists of gathering details of the onset of the first phobic episode, past history of other phobias, childhood anxiety, current symptoms, and triggers. Current symptoms usually include intense anticipatory worrying and autonomic activation including increased heart rate, sweating, tremor, hyper-alertness, an inability to nap or sleep, or a hesitancy to play at full speed or with full contact. The phobic anxiety is usually triggered just before travel or competition but can be more intense if the match is more important, the athlete has not been playing well, or there are off-field stressors like family or financial concerns.

Travel phobias are usually easy to treat with behavioural strategies and targeted medications. Athletes typically use the relaxation breathing techniques described earlier (Section 1.2.2). These are more effective if they have been practised daily and used routinely. After boarding the plane they take their seat and with eyes closed, breathe in through the nose for a count of 4, hold for 7, and breathe out for 8 through the mouth repeated eight times followed by easy, quiet breathing. If activation occurs at any time during travel they can use a breathing routine of in through the nose for a count of 4, out through the mouth for 4, then in for 4 and out for 8, then in for 4 and out for 12. If these techniques are not effective then the athlete can use nasal hyperventilation which can be done quietly for three 20-second sets each followed by a very long clearing breath. Short-acting benzodiazepines like lorazepam or alprazolam can also be used and taken 30–60 minutes prior to departure. For longer flights (6 hours or more), some phobic athletes prefer to sleep and may take higher doses of benzodiazepines or even a hypnotic such as zopiclone.

Re-injury phobias are more difficult to treat and usually require graduated exposure and desensitization. It is important to make sure the athlete fully understand their injury and surgery and the healing/recovery process. Any specific or general doubts are fully discussed with the medical team and reassurance is given where needed. In collaboration with the medical team a step-wise plan of increased practice duration, intensity, and contact is created. Fear, apprehension, and doubt are monitored. Sleep, soreness, swelling, and pain are also assessed regularly and any concerns are discussed. As activity and intensity are increased, the athlete usually becomes more confident and relaxes into automatic movement patterns. After first contact most report a great sense of relief when re-injury does not occur. It is important to inquire if performance is improving steadily to pre-injury levels as 10–25% of those with serious injuries (e.g. Achilles tendon rupture, anterior cruciate ligament tear, or joint dislocation) will have a permanent post-injury performance decrement. Medication is not typically needed although a low dose of short- or long-acting benzodiazepines (diazepam 5 mg, lorazepam 0.5 mg, or clonazepam 0.5 mg) can be used as a muscle relaxant in collision sports. Pain is managed in typical ways with local treatment and anti-inflammatories. If insomnia occurs then a hypnotic can be used.

1.3.2 Social anxiety

Social anxiety often starts as performance anxiety but as time passes and sports performance is inhibited, then anxiety in other social or performance situations develops. Social anxiety often begins in childhood but at that stage may not be severe enough to interfere with socialization or learning. It will often worsen in later school years as performance pressures rise. In schoolwork and sports, a discrepancy between performance and ability level is often seen. Symptoms typically include slowed concentration and memory retrieval, conscientiousness, overthinking, distractibility, and nervousness.

Assessment focuses on symptoms and thought patterns during the situations that provoke most anxiety. Specific phrases that are thought or spoken are recorded exactly (such as 'I'm going to choke', 'I'll look stupid', 'I'll make mistakes and be taken out', 'I'll embarrass myself', 'or I'm going to say something dumb') so that a countering phrase can be created. Recording these phrases in writing and their associated emotions and actions promotes increased self-awareness and cultivates a sense of mastery.

Treatment is usually with a combination of cognitive behavioural therapy (CBT) augmented by role play (to review recent awkward interactions and practise future ones) and medication. Strong positive phrases are crafted to counter the negative thinking and self-talk (e.g. 'relax and take it easy' and 'Be yourself and show confidence'). Athletes are encouraged to seek out social interactions with those they are more comfortable with and to tell them about their social anxiety and ask for support. Typical medications are SSRIs or SNRIs with adjunctive buspirone or short-term, low-dose benzodiazepines as needed. Relaxation breathing is also encouraged before the anxiety-provoking situations and long, easy clearing breaths through pursed lips can be used during these periods.

1.3.3 **Generalized anxiety**

Generalized anxiety typically occurs in adults in two types. One is the evolution of an overanxious child into a generally anxious adult and the other is adult onset following a significant loss or major trauma. Generalized anxiety may first appear to be performance anxiety restricted to sports but with time it becomes clear that it is more widespread. These athletes are very active thinkers, results oriented, often shy and perfectionistic, and commonly overanalyse their performance, especially focusing on mistakes and defeats rather than successes or achievements.

There are usually broad-based worries about all aspects of life including family, friends, school or work, sports, and hobbies. The most common symptoms are excessive worrying, negative thinking, pessimism, and increased arousal with increased heart rate and breathing, tremulousness, muscle tightness, unsteadiness, light-headedness, flushed face, decreased visual acuity, and increased sweating. Assessment requires a detailed past history from childhood and a documentation of current symptoms and control strategies. It is important to make sure the athlete is sleeping and is not using either alcohol or stimulants to excess. High-dose caffeine (more than 500 mg a day) in some athletes can raise baseline anxiety and can be a treatment barrier. The Beck Anxiety Inventory or the Hamilton Anxiety Rating Scale can be used and will often identify the generalized nature of the problem as well as being helpful for tracking improvements with treatment. It is important to make sure that co-morbid ADHD or a depressive disorder is not present.

Treatment typically requires a combination of individual therapy using cognitive behavioural/motivational enhancement strategies, relaxation and attention training, and medication. Individual sessions focus on reducing anxious activation and futuristic fear-based thinking. This is done by narrowing attention so that a feeling of being 'in the moment' is encouraged. Sometimes positive phrases that represent this are repeated ('my time—this space'). Grounding techniques described earlier in Section 1.2.4 are learned and inserted into daily routines. Kinetic chain activation with slight rhythmic movements and enhanced feel are included. An important concept to grasp is that activation of automatic brain networks involving breathing, feel, rhythm, sound, and sense can deactivate excessive thinking and worrying and reduce the associated negative emotions such as fear and doubt. Medication options include an SSRI/SNRI but often at higher dosages and more often with adjunctive low-dose benzodiazepines. Weight gain may be an issue and venlafaxine may be preferred for this reason. If ADHD is present, care must be taken to avoid the increased anxiety that can occur with short-acting stimulants at higher dosages.

1.3.4 **Panic disorder**

Panic tends to have an abrupt onset without an obvious trigger but often in crowded, closed spaces, while driving, or during periods of exertion. Once a single panic attack has occurred then it is far easier to have further episodes. Triggers include going back to the same place or engaging in the same activity as the first attack or any moderate activation of cardiovascular functioning. It is also common for the first episode to develop during high-stress periods. Occasionally attacks are triggered by cannabis use and can persist for weeks or longer even after use is discontinued.

There is often a past history of social or generalized anxiety and a family history of worrying or anxiety. Symptoms usually occur in those with high baseline anxiety who have high performance standards.

Panic occurs in 1–3% of larger groups of athletes per year. Sometimes there is an unidentified learning or attention problem that may explain ongoing apprehension and fear.

Typical symptoms are intense and include a fear of dying or losing control, rapid heart rate with palpitations, breathlessness/air hunger/hyperventilation, dizziness, blurry vision, and derealization. Some individuals seek emergency medical attention thinking they are having a heart attack or stroke. Anticipatory worrying and social withdrawal with rumination and fear are also common. Crowded places are avoided and even driving can be affected for fear of having an episode.

Assessment requires a detailed history of the first and subsequent episodes and the adjustments made as a result of these. Current and past stress levels must be documented as well as past adjustment, social anxiety, or generalized anxiety. A history of substance misuse must be taken to ensure that high-dose stimulants or heavy drinking are not involved. Short-acting stimulants (prescribed or not) can block the resolution of panic attacks once they have become engrained.

Panic attacks need to be aggressively treated as soon as they occur with a combination of stress control or relaxation training, CBT, and medication. The breathing techniques described earlier (patterned, clearing, controlled hyperventilation) should be practised several times daily. Often nasal hyperventilation followed by patterned relaxation breathing (4–7–8) is the most effective. Once an individual realizes that they can produce many of their panic symptoms by controlled hyperventilation and then manage them with patterned or clearing breathing, then they begin to regain confidence. Becoming aware that symptoms are not life-threatening and result from the effects of respiratory alkalosis reduces worry and promotes relaxation. It is also important to have an active dialogue about fears (dying, losing control, going mad) and some of the more unusual symptoms such as blurred vision, derealization, tinnitus, or dizziness.

Medication options include benzodiazepines in a fixed schedule and at higher dosages initially. Long-acting clonazepam 0.5 mg twice a day and 1 mg at bedtime works well unless there are problems with daytime sedation, mental slowing, or decreased reaction time. If so, then the daytime dosages can be halved and taken two or three times during the day. Alternatively, a trial of regular alprazolam 0.5 mg twice daily and 1 mg at bedtime may prove less sedating. If the panic symptoms can't be reduced in frequency or severity with therapy and benzodiazepines then a trial of an SSRI/SNRI is warranted.

When heavy alcohol or regular or heavy stimulant use is identified, the dosages must be reduced. It is common for adult athletes to use alcohol to unwind, not knowing that this can interfere with sleep quality. They may also use stimulants such as caffeine, nicotine, or amphetamines to help study, to support training or practice, and to combat fatigue. Dosages of caffeine above 500 mg a day are a concern. Other strategies to raise energy levels can be learned, for example, three 60-second bursts of cardiovascular activity, nasal hyperventilation, mini stretch breaks, or power naps.

1.3.5 Obsessive–compulsive disorder

Major classificatory systems include OCD in the group of anxiety disorders. While anxiety is a common and distressing feature of this condition, the central features are obsessions and compulsions. The disorder is thought to affect 1–2% of the adult population (lifetime prevalence) but seems less common in sport.

Obsessions may take the form of thoughts or ideas and images. The sufferer recognizes that these are his/her own (so-called ego-syntonic). The experiences are recurrent, entering the sufferer's mind repeatedly. They are also intrusive, unwanted, and unpleasant. As a result there are attempts to resist but these cause anxiety and are invariably unsuccessful. Resistance breaks down and the thought recurs.

Examples might include thinking that whatever you think will come true; a thought that you might shout out a blasphemous phrase in the middle of a religious ceremony; and a thought or images of jumping in front of a train or from a tall building.

Compulsions are actions carried out repeatedly and usually in a stereotyped manner. The behaviour is usually without purpose. The sufferer recognizes this but is nonetheless compelled to complete the act or else to experience severe anxiety often as a result of fearing that some unlikely harm will result.

Examples might include repeatedly checking the gas taps on the cooker for fear of causing an explosion, and multiple and repeated hand-washing for fear of being contaminated with germs.

Symptoms are usually readily described when an enquiry is made but may not otherwise be volunteered. The symptoms amount to a disorder when they are present on most days for a sustained period of weeks and when they cause distress or interfere significantly with functioning. They can be exceptionally time-consuming and interfere significantly with daily activities.

Obsessional and compulsive symptoms can also occur either as normal phenomena or secondary to another condition. If this is the case then the other condition (a mood disorder or psychotic condition, for example) is the primary diagnosis.

Many sportspeople use highly ritualized behaviours as part of the preparation for performance. Superficially these may resemble stereotyped compulsions. Anxiety may be present especially if the athlete is unable to carry out the act. It is also common for sportspeople to experience thoughts and perform rituals driven by superstitions about their performance (lucky kit, talismans, mascots, etc.) and to experience anxiety if this is prevented. However, these behaviours are likely to be both functional (they enhance performance) and not pervasive (they are present only in the sporting arena). If there is extension into other areas or interference with other activities then OCD should be considered. If the rituals and thoughts start to impair performance then interventions (suitable for milder forms of OCD) can be considered even if a full OCD syndrome is not present.

When functional impairment and distress is relatively mild then CBT is the preferred treatment option. This would include offering the specific technique of exposure with response prevention. This is a form of exposure therapy where the subject is exposed to the feared situation but prevented from performing any ritual or compulsive act until anxiety abates.

When functional impairment is at a moderate level, a choice of either CBT or drug treatment with an SSRI such as sertraline or fluoxetine can be offered. Drug treatment can also be offered when milder symptoms do not respond to CBT. In severe cases, CBT and drug treatment should be offered as a combination.

Table 1.1 Common types of anxiety disorders		
Disorder	Symptoms	Onset and duration
Adjustment anxiety	Overthinking, analysing, worrying, comparing, nervous, tremulous, poor sleep, fatigue, irritability, disappointment, embarrassment	Rise in competitive level, injury, reduced or limited playing time Lasts weeks to months
Specific phobias	Fear of flying. Worry about crashing. Moderate–severe somatic anxiety (palpitations, sweats, tremor, short of breath, nausea, dizziness, and flushing) Fear of re-injury with worry about contact, falling to the ground, running at full speed, turning abruptly, getting hit, heading the ball, etc. Mild somatic anxiety and a myofascial guarding reflex	Often triggered by extreme turbulence or emergency landing. Often during high-stress periods Lasts hours to a day Re-injury fear is more common after serious injury with surgery and prolonged rehabilitation Lasts days to weeks
Social anxiety	Worry about fitting in, inadequacy, awkwardness, making mistakes, and being judged. Somatic anxiety including palpitations, sweats, lightheaded, restless, flushing, and feelings of unreality and detachment. Performance anxiety with thought stoppage, word finding difficulty, extreme self-consciousness, and stuttering	Often arises in early school years but becomes more prominent in high school. Seen in school, sports, social networks, family interactions, and public appearances Lasts years to decades
Generalized anxiety	Difficulty concentrating, poor memory, mind goes blank. Somatic anxiety including restlessness, fatigue, irritability, muscle tension, and sleep disturbance	Onset in adolescence or young adulthood and often preceded by separation, abandonment, and/or bedtime fears Lasts years to decades
Panic	Thoughts of losing control, dying, or going mad. Severe somatic anxiety (palpitations, sweats, tremor, short of breath, nausea, dizziness, and flushing) Difficulty focusing and an urge to flee or avoid trigger situations	Onset in late adolescence and young adulthood and is commonly associated with pre-morbid social or generalized anxiety and agoraphobia Lasts from weeks and months to years
OCD	Intrusive thought or images. Compulsions. Attempts to resist cause moderate–severe anxiety	Onset often in childhood or adolescence Can last for months to years

Case study 2: generalized anxiety with co-morbid attention deficit and depressive disorders

A 19-year-old baseball player developed increasing anxiety following a setback in his rehabilitation from ulnar collateral ligament surgery 4 months before. He had been overly aggressive in his throwing programme, trying to return too quickly. He complained of constant worrying about his sports future and intense social anxiety.

Assessment: a detailed history revealed increasing social and performance anxiety over several years. This had increased when he started playing at a higher level and transferred to a new high school following the divorce of his parents. He worried about fitting in and about his grades, family, and future. He reported always being behind in his school work because of disorganization and procrastination. He described trouble focusing on his studies and felt he performed below his academic potential. When discussing his parent's divorce he became upset saying that since his parents separated he had moved from his old neighbourhood and begun to feel sad most days. He lived primarily with his mother and a younger brother. He resented visiting his dad who was often critical of his sports performance. Formal assessment, including a family interview with both parents, revealed undiagnosed attention deficit disorder (inattentive type), generalized anxiety, and dysthymic disorder. Collateral meetings with his mother and father revealed lingering conflicts and unresolved emotions over the family separation and move. There was no history of alcohol, tobacco, caffeine, or other drug use.

Intervention: he was seen individually on a weekly basis for 6 weeks. The initial focus was on his surgery and rehabilitation and fears of missing an opportunity to play baseball in college. He was connected with an athletic trainer/strengthening coach to supervise his rehabilitation. As these sessions progressed his confidence improved.

To address his inattention, disorganization, and procrastination, he was started on long-acting amfetamine salts with an additional dose of a short-acting drug for longer days. His focus and attention improved in the classroom. He also found a school-based tutor and they met once a week to help plan his study time.

For his anxiety and insomnia he was shown relaxation and grounding techniques. In addition, he had treatment with escitalopram 5 mg initially but increased to 10 mg after 3 weeks and finally to 15 mg a month after that.

The combination of medication and therapy resulted in a gradual reduction of his anxiety and led to a more open discussion of his sense of loss of his family and old neighbourhood. Individual meetings with his mother and father and a joint meeting with his younger brother were scheduled. These were productive and clarified the unresolved family conflicts and emotions. Consequently, several sessions with the father and his sons were held where some old resentments were discussed and plans for new approaches to family life were developed. He continued with stimulant medication and escitalopram and was able to resume baseball in time for the next season.

1.4 **Summary and conclusions**

Anxiety disorders are the most common mental disorder seen in sport and occur in two distinct groups—adjustment anxiety and primary anxiety disorders (see Table 1.1). Adjustment anxiety develops in relation to an identifiable stressor and usually last for

Table 1.2 Primary anxiety disorders			
Disorder	Screening and assessment	Medications	Therapy
Adjustment	Stressors Stress reactions Substances	Benzodiazepines Short-term, lower-dose SSRI/ SNRIs	CBT, motivational enhancement, stress control, relaxation training
Specific phobias	Childhood fears Trauma and loss	Benzodiazepines— short term or occasional use	Systematic desensitization, stress control, relaxation training
Social performance	Perfectionism Reacting to mistakes and losses	SSRIs, SNRIs Buspirone Benzodiazepines, hypnotics	Role play, CBT, relaxation, grounding
Generalized	Separation anxiety and phobias in childhood Trauma and loss Substance misuse	SSRIs, SNRIs Buspirone Benzodiazepines, hypnotics	CBT, relaxation, grounding
Panic	Generalized anxiety, social anxiety, learning disorders Substance misuse	SSRIs, SNRIs Buspirone Benzodiazepines, hypnotics	CBT, stress control
Obsessive–compulsive disorder	Obsessions, compulsions, rituals, superstitions. Nature and extent of functional impairment	SSRIs	CBT, exposure with response prevention

weeks to months. Primary anxiety disorders are more chronic and their origins can be traced into childhood or to a specific traumatic event. Adjustment anxiety is often complicated by substance misuse and primary anxiety is often seen with co-morbid attention deficit/learning and depressive disorders. The treatment approach to each is similar (see Table 1.2) and works best if a collaborative care model with the medical team (trainers, strength and conditioning staff, physicians, chiropractors, physiotherapists, etc.) and coaches is utilized. This is easier if mental health providers are available on-site during training and practice and/or prior to competitions. Brief or time-limited therapy models such as behavioural, cognitive behavioural, and/or motivational enhancement work best. If the natural social support groups around an athlete are utilized (i.e. family, friends, teammates, and coaches) and the cases are identified early, then the outcomes are excellent. Medication can often be used in lower dosages and for shorter periods of time when combined with social support and therapy. Finally, sleep and stress control is critical to good care and outcomes.

Further reading

Baron, D.A., Reardon, C.L., and Baron, S.H. (2013). *Clinical Sports Psychiatry*. Oxford: Wiley-Blackwell.

Glazer, D.D. (2009). Development and preliminary validation of the Injury-Psychological Readiness to Return to Sport (I-PRRS) scale. *J Athl Train* 44(2):185–9.

Glick, I.D., Stilman, M.A., Reardon, C.L., and Ritvo, E.C. (2014). Managing psychiatric issues in elite athletes. *J Clinic Psychiatry* 73(5): 640–44.

Grand, D. and Goldberg, A. (2011). *This is Your Brain on Sports: Beating Blocks, Slumps & Performance Anxiety*. Indianapolis, IN: Dog Ear Publishing.

Lardon, M. (2008). *Finding Your Zone: Ten Core Lessons for Achieving Peak Performance in Sports & Life*. New York: Penguin Group Publishing.

Loehr, J. and Schwartz, T. (2003). *The Power of Full Engagement: Managing Energy, Not Time is the Key to High Performance and Personal Renewal*. New York: Free Press.

McDuff, D.R. (2012). *Sports Psychiatry: Strategies for Life Balance & Peak Performance*. Washington, DC: American Psychiatric Publishing.

Monsma, E., Mensch, J., and Farrol, J. (2009). Keeping your head in the game: sport-specific imagery and anxiety among injured athletes. *J Athl Train* 44(4):410–17.

Porter, K. (2003). *The Mental Athlete: Inner Training for Peak Performance in All Sports*. Champaign, IL: Human Kinetics.

Reardon, C.L. and Factor, R.M. (2010). Sport psychiatry: a systematic review of diagnosis and medical treatment of mental illness in athletes. *Sports Med* 13:961–80.

Tofler, I.R. and Morse, E.D. (2005). *Clinics in Sports Medicine: The Interface between Sport Psychiatry & Sports Medicine*. Philadelphia, PA: Elsevier Saunders.

Visek, A.J., Harris, B., and Blom, L.C. (2013). Mental training for youth sports teams: developmental considerations & best practice recommendations. *J Sport Psychol Action* 4(1):45–55.

Chapter 2

Managing the anxiety of performance

Kate Goodger and Sarah Broadhead

Key points

- Competitive or performance anxiety is a specific type of anxiety associated with the perceived threat of performing a task under pressure.
- Whilst competing in sport, athletes can experience psychological states ranging from one of 'choking' where anxiety significantly inhibits performance to 'flow' where actions are effortless, easy, and feel natural.
- Levels of attention can be influenced by an athlete's mental state under pressure.
- Athletes can decide the optimal mental state in which they would like to train and compete and seek help to achieve that state.
- A number of techniques are available to help athletes attain their optimal mental state. Each has its pros and cons and an evidence base.

2.1 Introduction

Overcoming obstacles and adversity is integral to the life of an athlete. Adversity may take the form of a setback such as an injury, or chasing down a lead against tough opponents. One of the major challenges for an athlete is overcoming that posed by his or her own psychological state and more specifically, the ability to overcome and manage pressure. Pressures are factors or combinations of factors that increase the importance of performing well. They may be real or exist primarily in the mind and perceptions of the athlete.

Sport has become a global industry with events such as the Super Bowl and the Olympics among the most watched events on the planet and evaluation is largely by binary criteria—winning or losing. An athlete's performance is judged (whether by themselves or others) and in turn, there are consequences (real or perceived) associated with the outcomes of performance. An athlete will believe they have something significant to lose or to gain. This is often described as a 'fear of failure' or 'fear of consequence'.

Anxiety associated with performance (commonly referred to as 'competitive anxiety' or 'performance anxiety') has been explored primarily via the applied practice and empirical research of sport psychology. It has been defined as 'an unpleasant psychological state in reaction to perceived threat concerning the performance of a task under pressure'. It is considered to be the most common source of situational stress in sport, and is related to the perceived 'ego-threatening' nature of the competition. The public scrutiny and evaluation in sport can mean that both participation and performance are strongly linked to an athlete's self-esteem and self-worth. Therefore, when working with an athlete it is important to understand the meaning of sport and performance for that athlete.

2.2 **Choking and flowing**

The impact of anxiety on athletic performance is individual and hence variable. In the same pressured situation one athlete may literally 'freeze' whilst another appears to thrive. Many colloquialisms have developed to describe how athletes can be affected. Some of these are described here with an overview of how the mental states that are associated with optimum performance can be achieved.

2.2.1 **Choking**

'Choking' is a colloquial term for the stress response that culminates in a significant drop in performance and which psychologically damages the performer. This is often dramatic, for example, when an athlete is leading, seemingly close to victory, their performance begins to deteriorate, and then cannot be recovered. It may happen as a single incident or occur over a more prolonged period leading to a sustained loss of form. The athlete may come to perceive themselves as a failure, unable to handle pressure, and a 'choker'. There is often great fear of being associated with this label.

Explanations of 'choking' have empirical support and focus on the relationship between increasing anxiety or pressure and attentional focus. Some explanations suggest it is the result of a situation raising both anxiety levels and self-consciousness about performing successfully. Consequently the athlete increases their attention on the execution of the skill through either increased conscious control or step-by-step monitoring of the execution. The result is close to paralysis of the ability to execute an action that is no longer automatic. An alternative explanation is that attentional focus is taken away from task-relevant cues such as the ball or an opponent to task-irrelevant cues such as worrisome thoughts. This creates a dual-task situation rather than the single-task situation that is optimum for performance execution. In these circumstances, the processing efficiency of the brain is compromised and performance deteriorates.

The sports psychiatrist can work across cognitive, emotional, attentional, and situational factors to help prevent an incidence of choking (see Section 2.3). After an episode of choking there are implications not just for future performances but also for the self-perception of the athlete whose identity is strongly associated with their sport. This can mean that there is significant work needed to achieve recovery once choking has been experienced.

Case study 1

A 20-year-old golfer was finding it hard to strike the ball in the same manner during competition as in practice rounds. She and her coach found it frustrating and confusing as she experienced increasing unpredictability in competition despite consistency in practice. In one competitive round in particular it was noted that performance progressively deteriorated throughout.

The golfer was assessed to be in a relaxed state when practising but was noted to perceive competition as threatening. In particular, she feared the potential consequences of letting down significant others such as her coach, family, and sponsors. This produced a profoundly anxious stress response that was associated with the observed drop in performance.

The golfer and coach worked with a sports psychiatrist to understand why competitions seemed so threatening. Using cognitive therapy techniques she was helped to see sport in a different perspective and no longer such an anxiety-provoking 'life-and-death' situation. This approach was combined with work to focus on the process of each golf shot with the aim of increased consistency and the ability to execute the same shot regardless of situation.

2.2.2 Clutch performances

At the other end of the continuum to choking are 'clutch' performances. These are performances where an athlete is seen to perform better under conditions of pressure. 'Big occasion' or 'game-changing moments' appear to facilitate an increment in performance.

Explanations include one or some of a combination of factors such as greater investment in effort and resources that heighten attentional focus and mental processing efficiency, increased motivation, and the athlete's positive appraisal of their ability to cope with the demands of the situation. Athletes may also perceive physiological symptoms of anxiety in positive terms, for example, as a state of arousal that can energize performance.

2.2.3 Flow

An optimal mental state for performance is often described as when an athlete is in 'the zone' or in a state of flow. Flow is 'to feel at one with what you are doing, to know you are strong and able to control your destiny at least for the moment, and to gain a sense of pleasure independent of results'. In this state, skill execution is fluid and effortless. Eight dimensions or components characterizing this state have been described:

- Challenge–skill balance—the task must be challenging yet the individual perceives they have the skills to meet the demands of the task

- Merging action and awareness—involves complete immersion or absorption in the task (a hallmark feature of flow)

- Clear goals and feedback—these provide self-assessment which can be intrinsically motivating, especially when feedback is positive and progress is made towards the goal

- Concentration on the task at hand such that execution feels automatic

- Sense of control—a sense of empowerment and perception of control over performance outcomes

- Loss of self-consciousness—so that the task is performed without fear, anxiety, or inhibition

- Transformation of time—sometimes this is associated with a loss of awareness or perception of time

- Autotelic experience—where there is full immersion in a task that is intrinsically rewarding.

2.2.4 **Ideal performance state**

Sport psychology practitioners work with athletes to optimize performance through the development of an ideal performance state (IPS). A systematic approach to attaining this state can be developed. This involves the combination of emotions, cognitions, and physiological parameters that support an athlete to achieve an optimum performance. The state is both individual and task specific and hence it varies from one athlete to another and from one sport to the next.

Hardy and colleagues have described a six-item framework of the variables that help to create the IPS. This can guide the sports psychiatrist in helping athletes develop the attributes and skills that underpin the state:

1. Foundational attributes such as:

    • personality traits

    • motivational orientations

    • athlete's beliefs

2. Psychological skills:

    • goal setting

    • relaxation

    • self-talk

    • imagery

3. Strategies for training and competition:

    • pre-performance routines

    • performance evaluations

4. Adversity coping skills and strategies:

    • solution-focused coping

    • social supports

    • appraisal skills

5. The IPS:

    • a description of what this is for a particular athlete

    • how to attain it

    • how to maintain it

6. The environment—comprising four elements that influence the IPS for that athlete. These span what helps achieve an optimal state and in contrast what leads to a dysfunctional state:

    • physical

    • social

    • organizational

    • psychological.

2.3 Attention and anxiety

Performances can be impaired as a result of the effect of anxiety on attentional control and focus. In states of anxiety (including in anxiety disorders), there is an enhanced tendency to attend to and process threatening stimuli and often an inability to disengage from processing threat-related stimuli. This leads to an increased perception of the extent of threats in the environment, and influences subsequent cognitive and emotional processes.

The practitioner can work with an athlete to develop their ability to focus attention on the present and on the relevant processes in the present. This reduces the distraction of cognitive intrusions associated with anxiety. Strategies that assist this approach include the following:

- Pre-performance routines
- The development and use of visual cues
- Cues during performance execution
- Refocusing cues and strategies when the athlete becomes aware that appropriate focus is being lost (e.g. an advertising hoarding or the manufacturer's name on the match ball)
- Planning to 'controlling the controllables' (i.e. devoting conscious attention to the things that are within an athlete's control and dis-attending to those that are not).

2.4 Techniques for managing performance anxiety

The techniques and approaches used to develop the emotional and mental skills for managing performance anxiety and other emotions are considered in this section. In many approaches it is helpful to be able to distinguish between emotional, cognitive, and behavioural symptoms and to be able to separate these from any underlying source of anxiety (symptoms versus causes).

2.4.1 Cognitive therapy

This mode of therapy is based on learning to recognize unhelpful patterns of thinking. The approach involves identifying multiple alternative ways of interpreting a situation and then testing out the most accurate and realistic interpretation. Successful therapy is reliant upon readiness to engage with the therapeutic process and willingness to challenge unhelpful thought patterns.

2.4.2 Behaviour therapy

This therapy focuses on behaviour patterns rather than thought processes. Normal animal reward systems in the brain mean behaviours are more likely to be repeated if they are rewarded. The intervention usually involves either removing an inappropriate or unhelpful stimulus or altering the response to a stimulus. This approach relies much less on the athlete engaging with the process. A coach is often best placed to reward or reinforce behaviours from an athlete and the sports psychiatrist can work collaboratively with the coach to employ behavioural strategies in the daily training environment and in competition.

Graded exposure is one form of behaviour therapy. This involves establishing a hierarchy of situations beginning with those that are only mildly anxiety provoking and building up to those that are associated with the highest levels of anxiety. The athlete is exposed to each situation in turn over a period of weeks and gradually learns to cope with the anxiety at each level.

Case study 2

A 25-year-old male athlete in a weight-controlled sport was finding it hard to stick to his diet plan. The sports psychiatrist met with the athlete and coach together to try and understand the problem. The sports psychiatrist had attempted to work with this athlete in the past but this had not been effective as the athlete did not like to talk about 'the things in my head'. The sports psychiatrist agreed with the coach that a behavioural approach was the best option in this case.

Behavioural techniques included sticking the plan on the athlete's fridge door and placing a tick by each meal as it was eaten. If the plan were completed by the end of the week there was a non-food-based reward. The coach and athlete also met regularly to monitor the plan and the coach offered praise when there was adherence to the plan. The athlete liked being accountable to the coach and reported finding it much easier to stick to his diet.

2.4.3 **Cognitive behavioural therapy**

This therapy is based on the concept that thoughts, behaviours, and emotions are interconnected so that breaking an unhelpful pattern in one area will influence the others in a positive way. This therapy looks at current problems rather than past events. This combined approach is more commonly used than cognitive or behavioural approaches on their own. There are a large number of therapists in mainstream healthcare and so this type of therapy is usually readily available if needed.

Case study 3

A 30-year-old female tennis player was competing in a tournament for the first time after a prolonged period of injury. She had been badly injured in the past and took many months to fully recover. The sports psychiatrist met with the athlete and discovered that she was having the following unhelpful thoughts, emotions, and behaviours:

- Thoughts—'I am not ready, everyone is going to be better than me'
- Emotions—anxious, fearful
- Behaviours—she overtrains in the weeks up to the event, putting strain on the injury.

The sports psychiatrist used cognitive behaviour therapy (CBT) to work on her thoughts and the behaviours. She learned to identify and challenge her thoughts and concluded 'I cannot do anything about the amount of training I have done since my injury. I have progressed at a rate that was safe for my body. If I push it too quickly I could get re-injured and miss the event altogether. I can only go and do my best and see what happens'. The sports psychiatrist also focused on her unhelpful behaviours (the tendency to overtrain) and she was encouraged to keep a diary to monitor how closely she was sticking to the training plan she had been given in the 2–3 weeks prior to competition.

By learning to identify unhelpful thinking and behaviour patterns quickly and readily and then to challenge and change them to more helpful ones, the athlete reported much lower levels of fear and anxiety before and during her next event.

2.4.4 **Relaxation techniques**

When the brain detects a threat, one of three mechanisms is activated by the sympathetic nervous system. These are the fight, flight, and freeze responses. The parasympathetic nervous system is responsible for subsequently calming the body back down to allow rest and recuperation in time for the next activation. Sustained anxiety produces a prolonged state of sympathetic activation and this has detrimental effects on the mind and body. Relaxation techniques have been developed to assist in reducing sympathetic activation and in achieving a less heightened state. Four popular relaxation techniques are described here.

Progressive muscle relaxation

This technique involves teaching individuals to relax muscles in a two-step process. Step one is to systematically tense a particular muscle group such as the neck and shoulders. Next, the tension is released and subjects are encouraged to notice how their muscles feel when relaxed from tension. The exercise progresses through different muscle groups usually starting from the feet and working upwards. By learning to tell the difference between a relaxed and a tense muscle, subjects can learn to return a muscle to its relaxed state.

This technique lowers overall tension and stress levels, and can be used during periods of increased anxiety. It can also be helpful for certain physical symptoms such as stomach aches and headaches and to improve sleep. Athletes are encouraged to practise twice a day in a non-stressful environment, often at home lying down. Sometimes reading a script of the technique during practice is helpful whilst others may play a recording of someone talking them through it. Spoken scripts are available as podcasts and written scripts can also be downloaded. As athletes become more skilled, they are able to use the technique when becoming aware of increased anxiety in other situations such as training or competition.

Breathing (diaphragmatic breathing)

When anxious, breathing can become more shallow and rapid, which in turn can make some anxiety symptoms worse. Diaphragmatic breathing will help to slow down the breathing rate and allow for deeper breaths.

The technique involves a series of smooth, slow, and regular breaths. Sitting upright is usually better than lying down or slouching, because it increases the capacity of the lungs to fill with air. It is best to 'take the weight' off the shoulders by supporting the arms on the side-arms of a chair, or on the lap. The process involves the following steps:

1. Take a slow breath in through the nose, breathing into the lower belly (for about 3–4 seconds)
2. Hold the breath for 1 or 2 seconds

3. Exhale slowly through the mouth (for about 3–4 seconds)

4. Wait 1–2 seconds before taking another breath.

About six to eight breathing cycles per minute is suggested to decrease anxiety. This will also regulate the amount of oxygen taken in and thus avoids the fainting, tingling, and giddy sensations that occur during over-breathing. Athletes can be encouraged to practise this technique daily and so be able to apply it when required.

Guided imagery

This method uses visualization/images to help the body attain a relaxed state. The usual process is for the subject to lie down with their eyes closed and be guided by the therapist to bring to mind a series of images. It is often combined with breathing techniques and muscle relaxation. Athletes may be asked to imagine a previous time when they were relaxed or to imagine themselves in a relaxed state. With practice, subjects can become sufficiently skilled to use the techniques without a therapist or guide and there are audio recordings and downloadable apps to help with this technique.

Biofeedback

Biofeedback uses precise instruments to measure an aspect of physiological activity such as brainwaves, heart rate, breathing, muscle activity, or skin temperature and then rapidly and accurately feedback this information to the user on their physiological state. The therapist explains how to read this physiological data and then assists the subject in learning some control over physiological functions such as heart rate and breathing rate. Over time the subject develops the ability to alter physiological functions without continued use of a measuring instrument.

2.5 Mindfulness

Mindfulness has become particularly popular among groups of athletes in recent years. Subjects learn to focus their mind on the present moment and on their immediate surroundings, rather than on either the past or the future. It encourages objective detachment from thoughts. Mindfulness allows the present moment to be seen clearly, without the need to fix things. This has clear links to the 'flow' state described in Section 2.1.3. Thoughts are allowed to drift in and out of the mind and the subject learns to see thoughts as just 'thoughts' and not something to engage or act on, or that has control over them and their mood.

This practice can often be complemented by yoga, meditation, or t'ai chi that helps bodily sensations to be noticed in even more detail.

2.6 The mind management model—chimp paradox

The 'mind management model' uses neuroscientific theories to provide a simple and practical explanation for how the mind works and how this influences human thinking, feelings, and behaviour. The model splits the mind into three systems:

System 1: a 'human' part of the brain that is rational, uses logical thinking, and looks for facts and evidence before acting

System 2: a more primitive 'chimp' part of the brain that uses emotional reasoning driven by survival instincts. The 'chimp' is quick to act and thinks independently from other parts of the brain giving us thoughts and feelings we may not want

System 3: a 'computer' which runs the brain's automatic functions (programmes). It tends to use pattern recognition and generates automatic thoughts and behaviours.

When working with this model, athletes will firstly be asked what they want to achieve and how they want to be in their home and sporting life. The framework is then used to explore emotions, beliefs, and behaviours, which systems these relate to, and to determine which are helpful or unhelpful in pursuit of their aims. Athletes are taught to recognize which system they are using in a particular situation, how to manage these systems, and how to choose the most effective system for a particular purpose.

Case study 4

A 19-year-old male had been competing in track athletics since the age of 6. He had been told he had injured his Achilles tendon and would miss the major event of the season. The sports psychiatrist met with him a number of times to understand what was happening in each part of his mind and noted that he expressed different thoughts and behaviours depending on which system was in charge at the time. Here are the responses seen from each system:

- Human: accepted the nature and extent of the injury, listened to the advice given and worked with the medical team and coaches to come up with a plan to return as quickly and safely as possible. Accepted that each day was a step closer to returning to full training and responded in a positive way with perspective.
- Chimp: reacted emotionally, seeing the injury as a catastrophe. The chimp experienced grief stages of denial, anger, depression, and bargaining (with coaches/physiotherapists to be able to train). These are all normal reactions for the chimp that lives only in the present and has no perspective. The injury is a threat to the ego, to self-esteem, and to survival of the athlete's identity.
- Computer: beliefs and behaviours stored here depend on the individual and their past experiences. The athlete had previously experienced a prolonged injury so his automatic thought was 'this will be extreme'. This view of himself, others, and the world is also stored in the computer. He saw himself as unable to cope and saw the world as unsupportive. This had a major influence on his response to the injury.

The chimp and computer were the dominant responses seen by the team, with the human only appearing infrequently.

The sports psychiatrist engaged the athlete by explaining the mind management model. The athlete was helped to understand their own human, chimp, and computer systems and taught to recognize which part of their mind was most active at a particular time. In this way, a plan was developed to manage each system.

This helped the athlete to remove unhelpful beliefs from their computer and be in the human part more often. He was able to follow the medical plans and keep the situation in perspective. He also reported feeling happier.

There are a number of techniques for managing performance anxiety, described earlier in this chapter. These techniques have been summarized in Table 2.1.

Case study 5

There is not always a right or wrong answer when deciding which intervention to use. However, some considerations that may aid this process are illustrated in this case study of a common problem.

Problem: a 24-year-old runner is anxious about an upcoming competition. It is the selection race for the World Championship later in the year. He is not sleeping well and becoming irritable with his coach and others around him.

Table 2.1 Overview of techniques for managing performance anxiety

Intervention	Pros	Cons	Evidence base
Cognitive behaviour therapy (CBT)	Can often be carried out over a small number of sessions, with results seen in a short space of time	Relies on learning skills and applying apply them outside of therapy Does not separate the person from the thoughts Subjects can experience a sense of failure if/when negative thoughts return	Large evidence base in non-athletic populations Frodi et al. (2010)—improvement in performance-related thoughts and behaviours Davis et al. (2009)—reduced salivary cortisol levels
Progressive muscle relaxation	Useful if the athlete can master the skill	Focuses on reducing symptoms rather than addressing root causes so may not be effective in all situations	Iqbal and Kluke (2010)
Breathing (diaphragmatic breathing)	Can be practised regularly and carried out anywhere	Tackles symptoms rather than causes	Schwab Reese et al. (2012)
Guided imagery	Can be carried out anywhere	Tackles symptoms rather than causes	Mousavi and Meshkini (2011)
Biofeedback	Once mastered can be carried out anywhere	Tackles symptoms rather than causes	Rice et al. (1993)
Mindfulness	Can use on a daily basis. Allows subjects to focus on the present	Not all athletes can develop this skill. Not always practical or desirable to stay focused on the present moment	Vollestad et al. (2012); Thompson et al. (2011)—significant reductions in task-related worries and task-irrelevant thoughts

Table 2.1 (Cont.)

Intervention	Pros	Cons	Evidence base
The mind management model—chimp paradox	Separate the person from unwanted feelings and behaviours. Less guilt when thoughts reappear Widely applicable as a generalizable emotional management process	Engagement necessary to learn the model and the associated skills	Limited academic research but many anecdotal accounts and endorsements (Victoria Pendleton, Chris Hoy, Ronnie O'Sullivan, and others) and objective measures of improved sporting performance (multiple world and Olympic titles)

Source data from Davis, H. et al., Salivary cortisol and mood reductions in Olympic athletes using cognitive behavioural methods, in Chang C.H., Handbook of Sports Psychology, Copyright (2009), Nova Science Publishers, Inc.; The Danish Journal of Coaching Psychology, 1(1), Frodi, A. et al., Experiences of cognitive coaching: A qualitative study, p. 1750–2764, Copyright (2010) Aalborg University and University of Copenhagen; International Journal of Sports Science and Engineering, 4(3), Navaneethan, B. and Soundararajan, R., Effect of progressive muscle relaxation training on competitive anxiety of male inter-collegiate volleyball players, p. 161–164, Copyright (2010) World Academic Press; International Journal of Academic Research in Business and Social Sciences, 1(3), Mousavi, S.H. and Meshkini, A., The Effect of Mental Imagery upon the Reduction of Athletes' Anxiety during Sport Performance, p. 342–345; Copyright (2011) Human Resource Management Academic Research Society; Journal of Sport and Exercise Psychology, 31(5), Otten, M., Choking vs Clutch Performance: A study of sport performance under pressure, p. 583–601, Copyright (2009) Human Kinetics, Inc.; Peters, S., The Chimp Paradox: the mind management programme to help you achieve success, confidence and happiness, Copyright (2012) Vermilion; Biofeedback and self-regulation, 18(2), Rice, K. et al., Biofeedback treatments of generalized anxiety disorder: Preliminary results, p. 93–105, Copyright (1993) Springer; Journal of Sport and Health Science, 1(2), Schwab Reese, L., Effectiveness of psychological intervention following sport injury, p. 71–79, Copyright (2012) Elsevier; British Journal of Clinical Psychology, 51(3), Vollestad, J. et al., Mindfulness—and acceptance-based interventions for anxiety disorders: a systematic review and meta-analysis, p. 239–60, Copyright (2012) John Wiley & Sons Ltd.

The sports psychiatrist will need a good understanding of the athlete to determine the following:

- Engagement—will the athlete engage with sessions? Does he want to discuss the problem and find a solution or does he want someone to solve it for him? If the latter, then behavioural techniques may be preferable. The sports psychiatrist can still work on building a relationship with the athlete and helping him see the benefits of opening up and talking.
- Skill level—if he is willing to engage, what is his level of skill in managing his mind? What is his level of commitment? If both are low, the chances of CBT or mind management working are also low. However, if his natural emotional skill level is low but his commitment is high, then he may still get some benefits.
- Underlying problems—is the cause of his anxiety related to significant underlying problems, for example, with self-esteem or other unhelpful values/attitudes/beliefs? If so, then the benefits of using an intervention that tackles the symptoms (relaxation techniques) may be more limited. The root cause will remain although some improvement will be noted. If the athlete wants to engage and work on their self-esteem or values then CBT or mind management can be considered.

In this case, the athlete was keen to engage with the sports psychiatrist and open up about the cause of his anxiety. It emerged after a few sessions that he had held a fundamental belief from childhood that you had to be good at everything to be liked. Failing at a competition was thus a major blow to his self-esteem. In discussions with his sports psychiatrist he opted to use the mind management model to challenge these beliefs. He worked on this daily over several weeks with regular and frequent support sessions with his psychiatrist.

After 6 weeks the athlete had shifted his values, beliefs, and how he viewed his sport. He worked on seeing sport and especially competition as a challenge and opportunity but not something that he would allow to determine his level of happiness. He would prepare as best he could and aim for selection but if he were not get selected he would reflect and work on what to improve for next time.

2.7 **Practical considerations in choice of intervention**

In addition to the practical points already considered around athlete engagement and existing skill level, there are some features of working in the sport environment that can impact the selection of intervention or approach:

- What psychological work has the athlete done previously?
- What did they find helpful or unhelpful about this work?
- What does the athlete currently do to prepare for training or competition? (Ask the athlete to guide you each stage of their pre-performance routine up until the competition starts.)
- What has been unhelpful prior to competitions in the past?
- At what stage of the year are you working with the athlete (e.g. preseason, or in the run-up to a major championship)?
- Is there sufficient time to achieve successful outcomes with an athlete before a major championship (such as being able to acquire a mental skill in a short time)?
- What is the best way for an athlete to practise their anxiety management skills; can this be developed with the coach in training?
- How can an athlete measure their progress in relation to managing anxiety?

Further reading

Baumeister, R.F. (1984). Choking under pressure: self-consciousness and paradoxical effects of incentives on skilful performance. *J Pers Soc Psychol* 46:610–20.

Beck, A.T. (1979). *Cognitive Therapies and the Emotional Disorders*. New York: Penguin.

Cheng, W.N.K., Hardy, L., and Markland, D. (2009). Toward a three-dimensional conceptualization of performance anxiety: rational and initial measurement development. *Psychol Sport Exerc* 10:271–8.

Davis, H., Baron, D., and Gillson, G. (2009). Salivary cortisol and mood reductions in Olympic athletes using cognitive behavioural methods. In Chang, C.H. (Ed.), *Handbook of Sports Psychology* (pp. 423–30). Hauppauge, NY: Nova Science Publishers, Inc.

Gyllensten, K., Palmer, S., Nilsson, E.K., Regner, A.M., and Frodi, A. (2010). Experiences of cognitive coaching: a qualitative study. *Int Coach Psychol Rev* 5:1750–2764.

Hardy, L., Jones, G., and Gould, D. (1996). *Understanding Psychological Preparation for Sport.* Chichester: Wiley.

Harmison, R.J. and Casto, K.V. (2012). Optimal performance: elite level performance in 'the zone'. In Murphy, S.M. (Ed.), *The Oxford Handbook of Sport and Exercise Psychology* (pp. 707–24). New York: Oxford University Press.

Hill, D.M., Hanton, S., Matthews, N., and Fleming, S. (2010). Choking in sport: a review. *Int Rev Sport Exerc Psychol* 3:24–39.

Iqbal, Y. and Kluke, D.A. (2010). Effect of progressive muscle relaxation training on competitive anxiety of male inter-collegiate volleyball players. *Int J Phys Educ Sport Sci* 5:44–58.

Jackson, S.A. and Csikszentmihalyi, M. (1999). *Flow in Sport.* Champaign, IL: Human Kinetics.

Mousavi, S.H. and Meshkini, A. (2011). The effect of mental imagery upon the reduction of athletes' anxiety during sport performance. *Int J Acad Res Bus Soc Sci* 1(3):342–5.

Otten, M. (2009). Choking vs. clutch performance: a study of sport performance under pressure. *J Sport Exerc Psychol* 31:583–601.

Peters, S. (2012). *The Chimp Paradox: The Mind Management Programme to Help You Achieve Success, Confidence and Happiness.* London: Vermillion.

Rice, K., Blanchard, E., and Purcell, M. (1993). Biofeedback treatments of generalized anxiety disorder: preliminary results. *Biofeedback Self Regul* 18(2):93–105.

Schwab Reese, L. (2012). Effectiveness of psychological intervention following sport injury. *J Sport Health Sci* 1(2):71–9.

Thompson, R.W., Kaufman, K.A., De Petrillo, L.A. Glass, C.R., and Arnkoff, D.B. (2011). One year follow-up of mindful sport performance enhancement (MSPE) for archers, golfers, and long-distance runners. *J Clin Sport Psychol* 5:99–116.

Vollestad, J., Nielsen, M.B., and Nielsen, G.H. (2012). Mindfulness- and acceptance-based interventions for anxiety disorders: a systematic review and meta-analysis. *Br J Clin Psychol* 51(3):239–60.

Yiend, J. (2008). The effects of emotion on attention: a review of attentional processing of emotional information. *Cogn Emot* 24:3–47.

Chapter 3

Mood disorders

Valentin Z. Markser, Alan Currie, and R. Hamish McAllister-Williams

---

Key points

- Mood disorders (depression and bipolar disorder) are both common and potentially serious.
- Whilst sports and exercise participation may be protective against becoming ill with a mood disorder, a sports environment also contains risk factors for depression and bipolar disorder.
- The stress of overtraining may lead to widespread symptoms including mood disturbance and depressive disorders.
- A diagnosis may be missed if no enquiry is made. This applies especially to manic/hypomanic symptoms in bipolar disorder. Screening tools and diagnostic schedules can help with diagnosis.
- Suicide is the most serious complication of mood disorders. Risks and protective factors should be assessed in every case.
- Good treatments are available that can be tailored to the individual.

3.1 Introduction

Mood disorders are common and potentially serious illnesses, and depression is the commonest form of these conditions. Worldwide, 350 million people are affected and depression is responsible for more 'years lost' to disability than any other medical condition. In recent years, the burden of disability associated with depression has increased. This may relate to increased recognition and diagnosis. It may also represent a true increase in incidence that results from the mental and social stress of modern performance-oriented societies. It is a misperception that being in a privileged position will protect against depression. This is most certainly not the case and mood disorders are seen across all groups of society, even the financially well-off and those in revered and respected positions, such as elite athletes.

Mood disorders are serious since they affect all aspects of a person's life and at times there is severe functional impairment. They can also be fatal and lead to suicide. There have been high-profile cases of elite performers who have died in this way. In addition, mood disorders are associated with an increased rate of fatal and non-fatal accidents and an increased risk of developing series physical illnesses such as diabetes or coronary heart disease. Indeed, depression increases an individual's risk of experiencing a heart attack by as much as smoking 20 cigarettes a day.

3.2 Classification and description of mood disorders

Mood disorders are divided into two categories: depression, sometimes referred to as unipolar depression or major depressive disorder (MDD), and bipolar disorder, which many used to call manic depression.

3.2.1 Depression

Depression is extremely common although estimated incidence and prevalence rates vary depending on the diagnostic criteria used. The illness can have an onset at any age with a median in the late 20s to early 30s. The point prevalence is around 3–5% of males and 8–10% of females. The lifetime prevalence is only about twice the point prevalence for two reasons. Firstly, depression is highly recurrent with as many as 80% of individuals who experience one episode having one or more further episodes. Secondly, for many people the illness runs a chronic course and 20% of episodes last for 2 years or more.

Depression frequently presents with comorbid physical illness or other psychiatric symptoms and conditions. High rates of depression have consistently been found in a range of chronic physical illnesses. Anxiety disorders are the commonest form of psychiatric comorbidity although substance misuse is also frequently seen. This may result from attempts to self-medicate but the relationship can also be reversed, as depression is a common complication of substance misuse.

A diagnosis of depression is made when a cluster of symptoms is present. The nature of the symptom cluster along with the number and duration of symptoms required to make a diagnosis is arbitrary. No account is taken of either aetiology or underlying pathophysiology when making a diagnosis although there is clear evidence of altered or abnormal neurobiology in those suffering from depression. The situation is complicated by the probability that depression is a heterogeneous condition with multiple aetiologies and underlying pathologies. However, diagnostic criteria, such as the International Classification of Disease version 10 (ICD-10) and the Diagnostic and Statistical Manual of Mental Disorders, fifth edition (DSM-5) do improve the reliability of a diagnosis (see Box 3.1 which describes questions to elicit the presence or absence of the nine symptoms that make up the DSM-5 criteria). Many authorities, including the National Institute for Health and Care Excellence (NICE) in the United Kingdom, recommend the use of DSM-5 on the basis that these are the criteria used to define populations of patients in treatment studies. Thus most of the evidence base to guide clinical management relates to individuals with this nature and severity of illness.

Depression can present in a myriad of ways. From a simple statistical perspective, DSM-5 criteria include nine possible symptoms (some of which can go in either directions, e.g. insomnia or over-sleeping) but only five of these nine are needed to make a diagnosis. Different people can have a different collection of five symptoms. A somatic syndrome with symptoms of early-morning wakening, diurnal mood variation (worse in the morning), weight loss, and diminished appetite and libido may be present.

Clinically it is likely that the most important issue is whether or not there is significant comorbid anxiety. The presence of anxiety is associated with a more severe overall presentation, a worse outcome, and can impact on the nature of the treatment needed.

3.2.2 **Bipolar disorder**

Bipolar disorder can be viewed as being on a continuum with depression at one end and manic episodes at the other. It is not as common as depression but prevalence does depend on where the diagnostic threshold is placed on the continuum. Typically it is considered to have a point prevalence of around 1–3% but there may be at least an equal number who have some mild bipolar symptoms although insufficient to make a formal diagnosis using current criteria. Interestingly, the rate of bipolar disorder is equal between men and women, unlike depression which is twice as common in women. The disorder is more commonly recurrent than depression and hence the lifetime preva-lence is similar to the point prevalence. Age of onset of bipolar disorder tends to be younger than depression, the peak being in the teens and early 20s. Both genes and environmental stress are risk factors and sleep disturbance and stress are common precipitants for an episode. Bipolar disorder is frequently comorbid with other condi-tions, especially anxiety disorders and substance misuse.

Bipolar disorder can present with depressive episodes like those described in the previous paragraph for (unipolar) depression but where psychomotor retardation and hypersomnia are more common. In addition, bipolar disorder may present with an elevated mood characterized by a symptom cluster that includes euphoria, irritability, inflated self-esteem, decreased need for sleep, increased talkativeness, distractibility, and disinhibited behaviour. If symptoms are severe, lead to impairment of function, and last a minimum of 1 week, then an episode of mania is diagnosed. Psychotic symptoms may also be present, for example, grandiose, persecutory, erotic, or self-referential delusions. When less severe, the episode is termed hypomania. If a patient has had at least one episode of mania then the diagnosis is bipolar I disorder. If there have only ever been episodes of hypomania (never mania) then the term bipolar II disorder is applied. This is the commoner type of episode and hence the commoner diagnosis.

DSM-5 defines hypomania as lasting for at least 4 days. The shorter the duration of elevated mood, the more caution should be used in making a diagnosis of bipolar disorder. In depression, some patients have diurnal variation in mood with the depres-sion being more severe first thing in the morning. In bipolar disorder, it is possible for the diurnal variation to be so marked that patients are depressed in the morning and hypomanic in the evening. To make matters even more complicated, patients can pre-sent with symptoms of both depression and hypomania/mania at the same time. Such episodes are called 'mixed'. These sound counterintuitive. However, they illustrate that the term 'bipolar' and its implication that depression and mania are the two 'poles' of an illness is an oversimplification. Indeed, mixed episodes are extremely common.

3.2.3 **Overtraining syndrome**

Successful training in power and endurance sports requires an intensity that leads to overload followed by appropriate recovery that allows adaptation to occur. Intense training takes the body into a temporarily overstressed state sometimes called over-reaching (OR). Periods of intense training (e.g. in a training camp) might then be followed by a period of lower intensity exercise and recovery. When training is going to plan, these rest periods result in super-compensation when the body becomes adapted to increased stress and performances improve. This is described as func-tional over-reaching or FOR. However, if rest is inadequate then recovery is impaired and performances can start to stagnate or decline. If this is severe or sustained then longer-term decrements may be seen with performances taking weeks or months to recover. Impaired performance like this with poor recovery when associated with other symptoms such as fatigue, muscle aches, and mood disturbance is usually termed over-training syndrome (OTS). There is no hard and fast distinction between non-functional OR and OTS and no evidence for any qualitative or quantitative differences in symptoms between the two states. Both involve signs and symptoms of psychological distress and/or endocrine disturbances in addition to decrements in athletic performance. Additional physical symptoms include loss of weight, disturbance of coordination, increased infections, and cardiac arrhythmias. Psychological symptoms include sleeplessness, low mood, irritability, loss of interest in training, lack of energy, and loss of appetite. Because the mechanisms underlying OTS are not fully elucidated it is at times referred to as an 'unexplained underperformance syndrome', especially in the United Kingdom. Depressive symptoms, whether by cause, effect, or comorbid association are extremely common in OTS.

3.3 **Prevalence**

3.3.1 **Depression**

Studies of the prevalence of depression in sport are limited but suggest that depression is as common as in the general population. Some studies suggest that depression occurs more frequently in high-performance sport whilst others report that depression is equally common when comparing elite/professional athletes and recreational sportspeople. Depression in athletes is more common in women (as it is in the general population) and more common in those experiencing pain (as it is in the general population).

Much depression may go unreported. There may be considerable stigma attached to a mental health problem in the world of sport. Depression can be misdiagnosed as a somatic disorder or may be missed in some cases of OTS. Depression may also result in self-treatment with alcohol, drugs, or gambling that can obscure the primary problem. It is also a misconception that in high-performance sport, individuals who are prone to depression will be selected out and not able to compete at a high level.

3.3.2 **Bipolar disorder**

In bipolar disorder, there is also limited literature to allow an accurate estimate of prevalence. This is likely the consequence of under-investigation rather than reflecting the absence of this condition in athletic populations. Stigma makes it difficult for individuals, perhaps especially elite sportsmen, to disclose a diagnosis and this makes under-recognition more likely. Further, bipolar disorder is frequently misdiagnosed in the general population because individuals are much less likely to present to healthcare professionals when elated than when depressed. For the active athlete there is an additional factor that may obscure a manic or hypomanic presentation as sports participation may allow high levels of activity to be normalized and excess energy to have an outlet that is not available to more sedentary individuals.

3.3.3 **Overtraining syndrome**

Endurance athletes are particularly prone to OTS, resulting from the difficulty in ensuring adequate recovery when training at high intensity for long periods. There are reports that at 60% of endurance runners have experienced at least one episode of OTS in their careers. Although evidence is limited it would also be expected that athletes who are closer to their physical and psychological limits would be more prone and that higher rates would therefore be found in elite performers. High rates of OTS are seen in young athletes as well as adults. A Swedish survey of 272 high school national standard athletes from 16 sports found some evidence for OTS in 37%, with the incidence being higher in individual sports (48%) compared with team (30%) and less physically demanding sports (18%).

OTS is commoner in those who have had a previous episode, with reports of 90% of swimmers with OTS experiencing at least one further episode in the next 3 years. It is not known whether this reflects a higher risk of OTS in some individuals or whether one episode makes another more likely. There is a parallel with depressive disorders where 80–90% of those who have had one episode will experience another at some point.

3.4 **Sport-specific risks for mood disorders**

There are several important points to consider when evaluating the risk factors for depression in sportsmen and women:

- Fame or material wealth are not protective factors and do not guard against developing depressive disorder. Depression can occur in any individual in any walk of life.
- Athletes are exposed to many physical and psychosocial stresses and high-performance sport has many demands that place enormous stress on individuals.
- Elite athletes do not participate in sport primarily to improve their health (as many recreational athletes do). This can mean that they take good health for granted which increases vulnerability to both physical and psychological ill health.

3.4.1 **Mental strength and psychological weakness**

Psychological techniques are an important tool of the elite performer and the marginal difference between winning and losing may be determined by mental strength in two competitors of matching physical strength and ability. However, these mental skills increase the ability to suppress physical and psychological concerns. This is compounded if depression is perceived by the athlete and those around them as a personal weakness. The stigma of depression coupled with lack of awareness or even denial of depressive symptoms will result in under-diagnosis and significant avoidable morbidity.

3.4.2 **Injury, pain, and unidimensional identity**

Physical injuries are a particularly important risk factor for depression in athletes, possibly more so in the young and when the injury is severe. Rates of depression in injured athletes as high as 20% have been reported and are associated with an increased incidence of suicidal thoughts and acts. Pain is an established risk factor for depression in the general population but a higher risk in athletes may result from the threat to an athletic career and to the athlete's identity. For the same reasons, many professional sportspeople are particularly prone to depression when their careers end. This emphasizes the need for athletes to avoid a unidimensional identity and to have other important elements in their lives.

3.4.3 **Autonomy**

The relationship that a high-performance athlete has with their coach, manager and support team is critical to success. However, it can also lead to dysfunctional psychological interactions, putting the athlete at risk of depression. An athlete can feel a loss of autonomy and disempowerment when their life is mapped out by others (agents, coaches, dieticians, physiologists, sports psychologists, and others). A situation can arise where praise only comes following success or improvements in performance. This is counter to the need that individuals have for unconditional support and affection from the important people in their life. If a relationship becomes entirely conditional upon a good performance then the athlete receives emotional support when it is needed least and is denied support or criticized at times of greatest psychological vulnerability. Guarding against this is a key element of prevention of depression in athletes.

3.4.4 **Expectation levels**

The spectators of many high-profile competitive sports are interested in winners, performances, and records. They participate in sporting achievement vicariously by means of identification and mechanisms of idealization. At the extreme, entire nations and political systems support the athlete generously for their own interests as for as long as s/he is successful. Unrealistic expectations of the individual from within him/herself and from others are created and this adds to the risk of depression and OTS. Idealization and unrealistic expectations can also make it harder for a depressed athlete to accept that there is a problem that needs addressing.

3.4.5 **Perfectionism**

Perfectionism as a personality trait (discussed in more detail in Chapter 7) can often be found in high-achieving individuals of many kinds including successful athletes. A degree of discontentment with performances and results is a requirement for a successful high-performance sports career. Younger athletes in particular may struggle with finding a balance between adaptive and maladaptive psychological responses to the challenges they have to meet throughout their career. For example a perfectionistic trait that includes not only striving for ever better performances but also persistently evaluating these performances in a negative and self-critical manner is likely to increase the risk of depression.

3.4.6 **Lifestyle**

The lifestyle of elite sportspeople may require frequent travelling and often across time zones. Sleep disruption can also result simply from sleeping in uncomfortable or unfamiliar environments. Sleep disturbance and jet lag have been identified as risk factors for both depression and bipolar disorder. Travelling can also lead to disruption of the athlete's normal support systems, separating them from friends, family, and partners.

Attempts to deal with sleep disturbance by using alcohol or hypnotics can exacerbate symptoms of depression. Their use will also impair sporting performance and increase the psychological pressures described previously.

3.4.7 Additional risk factors

Additional factors include the misuse of anabolic steroids that are associated with both depression and mania. Previous head injuries are also a risk and the prevalence of depression in players of American football who have experienced three or more concussions is more than double that of those who have only been concussed once.

3.4.8 Aetiology of overtraining syndrome

Most cases of OTS have a multifactorial aetiology although the salient factor is intensity of training and/or decreases in quality or amount of recovery. There is evidence for a 'dose–response' relationship between training intensity and OTS. Other triggers include monotony of training, too many competitions, inadequate nutrition, physical illness such as infections, personal problems, emotional stress in other areas, sleep disturbance, altitude exposure, and heat stress. There is thus a significant overlap with factors known to be relevant in the aetiology of depression.

The onset of OTS is usually insidious over weeks or months and linking changes in training and other stressors to the onset of the syndrome can be difficult. What is currently unknown is why some athletes develop OTS and others don't when the intensity of their training is increased. It could be that these additional factors go some way to explaining this variance and this has implications for the treatment and support that should be offered.

Whether or not OTS and depression overlap clinically, there is a high degree of overlap in risk factors and vulnerability that at the very least makes depressive comorbidity more likely in cases of OTS.

3.5 Diagnosing depression

Many depression screening tools are available. Sports-specific severity rating scales have been developed and these relate established diagnostic criteria to the important elements in the life of the individual being assessed—in this case a life of sport. So, for example, rather than simply asking if there has been a change in level of interest and enjoyment in things generally, it may be more appropriate to explore any change in interest in sport—is there still enjoyment from a good training session or performance? Similarly, when assessing concentration ask about the ability to maintain focus and concentration during training and competition.

There are many self-rated screening tools. Whilst these are easy to use because a clinician is not needed, they are either not sensitive enough to pick up all cases or have acceptable sensitivity but poor specificity with up to 50% of those who screen positive not actually suffering from a depressive disorder. Differentiating between those that do and those that do not requires the expertise of a clinician. Thus, as far as screening is concerned, the important issue is to have a high index of suspicion of the possibility of depression and to seek an appropriate clinical review. Box 3.1 suggests how screening questions can be used that integrates with DSM-5 criteria for depression.

Box 3.1 Screening and diagnosis of depression

Screening (recognition) and diagnostic questions for depression
Ideally screening questions for anxiety disorders should also be used due to the high prevalence of co-morbid depression and anxiety.
1. Screening questions for depression:

- Have you been consistently depressed or down, most of the day, nearly every day, for the past 2 weeks?
- In the past 2 weeks have you been less interested in most things or less able to enjoy the things that you used to most of the time?

If yes to either question, proceed to diagnostic questions for current major depressive episode.

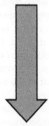

2. Diagnostic questions for current major depressive episode: Over the past 2 weeks when you felt depressed or had loss of interested/pleasure:

- Was your appetite decreased or increased nearly every day? Did your weight decrease or increase without trying intentionally? (If yes to either; code as yes)
- Did you have trouble sleeping, or have you been over-sleeping, nearly every night?
- Did you talk or move more slowly than normal or were you fidgety, restless, or having trouble sitting still almost every day?
- Did you feel tired or without energy almost every day?
- Did you feel worthless or guilty almost every day?
- Did you have difficulty concentrating or making decisions almost every day?
- Did you repeatedly consider hurting yourself, feel suicidal, or wish that you were dead?

If five or more 'yes' answers (including low mood and/or loss of interest/pleasure) are given (appetite/weight questions count as one question), and the symptoms are causing significant distress or impairment in social, occupational, or other important areas of functioning (e.g. sporting performance), then a current major depressive episode can be diagnosed.

Anxiety symptoms increase the likelihood of detection of psychiatric illnesses, as they are often obvious even to an untrained observer. However, as these symptoms are more obvious they can obscure an underlying condition such as depression. It is important to explore depressive symptomatology when anxiety is present and to clarify the primary diagnosis since there are differences in treatment recommendations, course, and prognosis.

3.6 Diagnosing bipolar disorder

Many patients with bipolar disorder have their illness unrecognized. Most commonly the condition is not recognized at all or is misdiagnosed as unipolar depression. This is because individuals are much more likely to seek help for low mood than if their mood is high. When hypomanic, an individual will often feel better than ever and this is not consistent with seeking medical help. However, it is important to distinguish the two conditions as the management of bipolar disorder is very different to that of depression. A useful rule is to ask carefully about symptoms of hypomania (e.g. lack of need for sleep, speeded thoughts, feelings of grandiosity, and disinhibition) at every presentation of an episode of depression. This can be done more formally using a self-completed screening tool such as the Mood Disorder Questionnaire (MDQ; Hirschfeld et al., 2000). Although there is some controversy about the best cut-off score to optimize sensitivity and specificity, it is worthwhile to carefully explore hypomanic symptoms in any patient who answers 'yes' to any of the questions. It would be essential to explore this in detail if there were a positive response to two or more questions or if significant problems had arisen in any area.

One of the key differentiations to make is between hypomania and simple wellness as this is not a distinction that has to be made when assessing depression. Another distinction that has to be made is from the positive thinking that athletes learn in order to be successful in high-performance sport. Factors to look for include whether the possible hypomanic symptoms are evident to others and to what extent they are out of character. If not then the individual may not be suffering from hypomania. It is also important to consider that anabolic steroids can lead to hypomanic and manic symptoms.

3.7 Diagnosing overtraining syndrome

Clinicians tend to diagnose what they are looking for. Such is the symptom overlap between OTS and depression that an elite sportsperson presenting to a psychiatrist might be diagnosed with depression but the same presentation to a sports physician or physiotherapist may be diagnosed as OTS. As there are no diagnostic tests to confirm or refute a diagnosis in either case perhaps the most important issue is to keep an open mind and focus on ensuring appropriate and helpful treatment regardless of the diagnostic label that is applied.

Biological findings have been used to try and identify markers of OTS to aid diagnosis and in particular to differentiate OTS and depression. These include cortisol, adrenocorticotropic hormone, prolactin, measures of oxidative stress, cytokines, measurement of plasma viscosity, blood lactate responses, and glutamine. However, to date, none are of sufficient clinical utility. The diagnosis is usually made after consideration of the training load, recovery periods (or lack of them) and their impact, and after other potential causes of the underperformance have been excluded. These include endocrine disorders such as thyroid conditions and diabetes, iron deficiency anaemia, infectious diseases, poor nutrition, or frank eating disorders such as anorexia nervosa. Not all guidelines emphasize the importance of screening for and excluding depressive disorders.

The close overlap between OTS and depression in terms of symptoms, aetiology, and biological and neuropsychological findings may be due to research that is confounded by individuals with depression being misdiagnosed as having OTS as well because the two are closely related physiologically and psychologically. Psychosocial stress can be a major factor in the development of OTS—a syndrome that commonly includes a depressed mood state. Elite sportspeople train hard. If they then experience a major life stress and develop low mood, is this depression or OTS? Depression itself is viewed as being a heterogeneous disorder with multiple aetiologies and pathophysiologies. In some ways OTS may simply be a variant with a very specific aetiological factor—overtraining. Whilst other factors, such as psychosocial stress, might exacerbate OTS, overtraining is *the* most important aetiological factor and it is this that distinguishes OTS from depression. An extra complexity is that OTS itself may be a risk factor for the development of depression and risk factors common to depression may explain some of the variance in OTS—why some athletes develop the syndrome whilst others who are training at the same intensity do not.

Mental illness attracts stigma and denial of psychological components to a presentation is common and not restricted to athletes. In addition, it is common for conspicuous psychiatric morbidity (especially anxiety and depression) to present with multiple, perhaps minor somatic complaints. In these circumstances there can be a long and fruitless search for a physical cause such as an infection that in the case of an athlete would 'explain' poor performance. However, even if evidence of an infection is found it can be hard to establish if this is a cause or a consequence of OTS or depression. In circumstances where somatic complaints are prominent, underlying psychological symptoms can be obscured. These include feelings of worthlessness, hopelessness and pessimism regarding the future, and suicidal ideation and planning. An enquiry about depressive symptoms is important or they may be missed and an appropriate aspect of management will be omitted.

3.8 **Further assessment**

3.8.1 **Investigations**

When assessing the depressed athlete it is important at an early stage to ensure that another condition is not being missed or misdiagnosed as a mood disorder. Some treatable conditions may cause mood disturbance (e.g. thyroid disorders or substance misuse) whilst others can complicate its course or exacerbate symptoms (such as poor nutrition or substance misuse).

Initial investigations are helpful in several respects. They will exclude or identify alternative causes of a disturbed mood, will help to evaluate co-morbid conditions and complications, and will provide a baseline where certain drug treatments are indicated. Suggested initial investigations are:

- Full blood count—to screen for, for example, anaemia and infections; raised mean cell volume can reveal harmful use of alcohol
- Urea and electrolytes, calcium—athletes may have significant abnormalities in electrolyte balance and calcium, particularly if there is a state of under-nutrition and poor hydration through neglect or if there is co-morbid disordered eating. Such imbalances might be enough to precipitate a mood disorder or prolong its course
- Glucose—to screen for diabetes and may guide treatment choices
- Proteins—are lowered as a complication of under-nutrition
- Thyroid function—disturbances may cause depression or mania. Lithium treatment may lead to hypothyroidism
- Lipid profile—because many antipsychotics are associated with the development of metabolic syndrome
- Liver function tests—especially if alcohol is suspected as a contributory factor or co-morbidity (look particularly for elevated gamma-glutamyl transferase)
- C-reactive protein—to screen for underlying inflammatory processes, for example, lupus
- Other tests as indicated, for example, urinary drug screen especially for cannabis and amphetamines and an ECG in drugs known to cause prolongation of the QTc interval such as tricyclic antidepressants and high-dose citalopram or escitalopram.

3.8.2 **Rating scales**

In any individual diagnosed with a mood disorder, the severity of the episode of illness needs to be assessed and then regularly reassessed to judge response to treatment. There is an important distinction between using a rating scale to make a diagnosis and measuring a condition where the diagnosis has been established. There are many rating scales available for the latter. Some are self-completed and others observer completed. The Quick Inventory of Depressive Symptoms (QIDS) comes in both forms (see http://www.ids-qids.org/index2.html). If there is close agreement between the self-rated and clinician-rated form at the outset then the self-rated form can be used on its own at subsequent reviews. The form comes in multiple languages. For mania, the Altman Self-Rating Mania Scale (ASRM: see http://www.cqaimh.org/pdf/tool_asrm.pdf) is useful. The simplest form of clinician-rated scale is the Clinical Global Impression scale (see Box 3.2). It rates the severity of the illness (depression or mania) on a seven-point scale and is quick, simple, reliable, and valid.

3.8.3 **Overtraining syndrome assessment**

An assessment includes taking a clear history to identify predisposing factors (family history of a mood disorder, personal and developmental history), precipitating factors (e.g. sleep disturbance), and perpetuating factors (ongoing stressors including physical comorbidity and unresolved psychosocial problems). Perhaps this is all the more important to emphasize if the initial assessment is undertaken by a non-mental health

Box 3.2 Clinical Global Impression (CGI) scales

CGI
Considering your total clinical experience, how severely ill has the patient been dur-ing the preceding assessment period?
1. Normal, not ill
2. Minimally ill
3. Mildly ill
4. Moderately ill
5. Markedly ill
6. Severely ill
7. Very severely ill

CGI—change
Considering the period immediately preceding this period of assessment, how much has the patient changed?
1. Very much improved
2. Much improved
3. Minimally improved
4. No change
5. Minimally worse
6. Much worse
7. Very much worse

Reproduced from Clinical Global Impression Scale, Guy, W., *ECDEU Assessment Manual for Psychopharmacology:* Publication, p. 76–338, Copyright (1976), reproduced under the Creative Commons License with permission from US Department of Health, Education, and Welfare, Washington, D.C.

specialist. It is important to fully explore the athlete's training history. Have there been recent changes in the training schedule? Have increases in training intensity been grad-ual and allowed for physical adaptation at each stage? Have periods of recovery been reduced? Has sleep disturbance due to, for example, travelling, led to reduced rest and recovery? Any unusual increases in training intensity or decreases in recovery may suggest the underlying aetiology is OTS. This aspect of the assessment is important for those mental health specialists who might have less experience of the sporting environment.

3.9 Management

3.9.1 Depression

A few depressed athletes may need a complete break from competition and possibly also from training and most will need some reduction in intensity of training to reduce both their psychological and physiological demands. Whilst a period away from sport may allow a sense of perspective to return, this will need to be an individual decision especially as a person whose entire sense of self is tied up with their sport may find it hard to be on the sidelines, even temporarily. Consideration can be given on how to include the athlete in team activities even if not in full training and this helps to instil hope and to maintain social contacts. A treatment plan can also include a graded return to activity as recovery progresses just as it would for an athlete with a physical injury. Indeed, treating the depressed athlete as an injured athlete has much to commend it and holds out hope that recovery is not just possible but a goal within reach and with a clear and shared path towards that goal.

The impact of training on depression and of depressive symptoms on performance both need consideration but in addition specific treatment must be offered. Many guidelines exist for the management of depression including those produced by NICE and the British Association for Psychopharmacology (BAP). These place importance on early identification and early treatment, recognizing that the duration of untreated illness correlates with non-response and a chronic course.

Treatments and interventions

For depression at the milder end of the spectrum (e.g. subthreshold and milder forms of DSM-5 major depression), non-specific support around anxiety and sleep management, guided self-help, and how to temporarily adjust sports training may suffice.

For those with more severe degrees of depression, specific psychological therapies (cognitive behavioural therapy (CBT) and interpersonal psychotherapy) and/or medication are warranted.

While there is some evidence that some antidepressants may be more potent than others, the relative difference in efficacy is small and so this is usually a minor consideration for the majority. The relative side effect burden of the various classes of antidepressants (and between individual drugs within classes), together with the presence of concurrent illnesses and additional medication are likely to be more important considerations.

In athletes, sedation can be a problem and more sedative antidepressants, such as tricyclic antidepressants and mirtazapine, are usually best avoided. If a patient has previously tolerated, and responded well to, a particular antidepressant then this drug should be considered first. In addition, if a close relative has responded well to a particular drug, there may be some value in considering that one. Otherwise there are few indicators of which patient will respond to which drug. Medication is discussed further in Chapter 10. Two important points, however, will be emphasized here. Firstly, antidepressants do not appear on the World Anti-Doping Agency's list of banned drugs. Secondly, athletes may attempt to stop and start treatment around competitions. This should be avoided if at all possible. Antidepressants need to be taken continuously and stopping runs the risk of discontinuation symptoms and relapse. If the athlete/coach is concerned that side effects are affecting performance, then this should be confirmed objectively and then an alternative drug can be considered.

Treatment effectiveness is assessed by monitoring a number of key symptom areas, such as mood, sleep, interest and concentration, as well as athletic performance. In addition it is important to assess treatment adherence and to monitor for the presence of side effects. The aim is for full remission of all symptoms. Patients who achieve partial remission with residual symptoms are at high risk of developing chronic problems and/or relapsing.

Lack of significant improvement after 2–4 weeks of treatment substantially reduces the probability of eventual sustained response. If a patient has made at least some improvement in this time then it is worthwhile continuing the same drug for 6–8 weeks.

If by 6–8 weeks there is only limited improvement, the diagnosis should be reviewed and maintaining psychosocial factors (including non-adherence) addressed. Possible next steps are to increase the dose of antidepressant or to switch to another drug (possibly from another class).

If there is no response to two cycles of this approach then more complex interventions are indicated. These may include an antidepressant drug and psychotherapy (CBT or interpersonal psychotherapy) together or combinations of antidepressant drugs. Specialist advice is recommended. As ever, it is better to do this sooner than later. Depression is bad for the brain, the rest of the body, and every facet of an individual's life including sporting performance, relationships (coach, family, and friends), work, and academic studies. The faster depression goes into remission the better.

Case study 1

A 52-year-old former professional cyclist described low mood during the winter months. In spring and autumn he worked abroad as a tour guide and felt mentally well. During this time he would cycle around 700 km a week. Around 4 weeks after returning home each autumn he experienced sleeplessness, depressed mood, became increasingly pessimistic in his thinking, was listless, and lacking in motivation. He tried to continue cycling in winter but the weather significantly curtailed his opportunities to ride.

He started cycling at a young age encouraged by his father who had been a professional cyclist. In his early 20s he became estranged from his parents, mainly due to conflicts with his mother. He won several national championships and competed in many classic cycling races including the Tour de France. During his racing career he had more than ten serious falls sustaining broken ribs on three occasions and two major concussions. As a rule he would continue racing the next day. At weekends or after cycling races he would experience loneliness and aggression and use alcohol regularly. After he retired from professional cycling he was easily bored and he was therefore very happy to become a tour guide with the opportunity to ride his bike regularly.

He presented for psychiatric treatment one winter when his low mood and sleeplessness were particularly bad. Initially, he agreed to take medication simply to get fit to cycle in the spring. By means of antidepressant medication (a selective serotonin reuptake inhibitor (SSRI)) and cognitive therapy he was more able to regulate his sleep and his mood improved.

He lacked emotional awareness and was not good at communicating his feelings. In this context his marital relationship was strained and his social contacts were restricted to cycling. He had few if any interests outside of sport and seemed to need to get recognition for his physical prowess and fitness. He also recognized that physical activity was therapeutic for him and he learned to use this during the summer months. Consultations were used to increase his motivation for longer-term psychotherapy.

In psychotherapy, he was able to explore and understand his motivation for intense physical exercise even after his professional career had ended. This helped him to develop alternative ways of coping with low mood during the winter months.

3.9.2 **Bipolar disorder**

The management of bipolar, like the disorder itself, is complex. Different treatments are used for the different phases of the illness and long-term prevention is the key issue.

There are not enough valid studies to make sport-specific treatment recommendations. Standard treatments can be used but with attention to tailoring the treatment and its tolerability to the individual and his/her circumstances.

Depressive phase

Many patients with bipolar disorder are treated with antidepressants when depressed. However, bipolar depression usually does not seem to respond to antidepressants—at least not to SSRIs. In addition, antidepressants are associated with an increased likelihood of a switch into mania and can cause an unpleasant syndrome of irritable dysphoria. As a result, most guidelines (including those from NICE and BAP) recommend that an antidepressant is *not* used as a first-line treatment. Unfortunately there are few medications with evidence of effectiveness in bipolar depression. These include quetiapine, lurasidone, lamotrigine, and the combination of olanzapine with fluoxetine. In general, these treatments are reserved for use by specialists.

Mania and hypomania

Hypomania and mania respond best to lithium, sodium valproate, or any antipsychotic (even when psychotic symptoms are not present). Lithium can be used even when exercising (see Section 10.3.2) but sodium valproate is associated with birth defects and must be used with great caution, if it is to be used at all, in women of child-bearing age.

Lifestyle management

Regular sleep patterns are important in managing mood disorders and especially bipolar disorder. Alcohol intake should be minimized as it disrupts normal sleep and may exacerbate and prolong mood symptoms.

Psychotherapy

Less is known about effective psychotherapy in bipolar disorder compared to its use in depression. The strongest evidence is for psycho-education provided on a group basis. This entails education about the nature of bipolar disorder, the importance of regular sleep patterns, the need for medication, and how to spot and manage early warning signs of relapse. Many find it helpful to develop a 'relapse template' that lists early signs and possible interventions that will halt the acceleration into a full relapse. These can include medication to support sleep, self-management of additional medications, for example, for early hypomanic symptoms, and rapid access to a specialist.

Case study 2

A 26-year-old professional basketball player was known to his team medical staff because of a recurrent depressive disorder. He had been treated on three occasions with fluoxetine with some response but found the drug hard to tolerate and complained of agitation and irritability. As a consequence he took treatment for the minimum period possible (usually around 4–6 months).

At the end of a busy season the team had a party over two nights. Although he was moderate with his alcohol consumption this did involve two consecutive late nights with limited sleep. He flew with his team from London to a tournament in Kazakhstan (a west to east time difference of 6 hours). The first match was late in the evening on the day after arrival. He played poorly and seemed to have difficulty concentrating. He had another late night (3 am) and slept poorly. The following evening there was a charity match followed by an official reception and another very late night. The next day was more relaxed and the team did some sightseeing.

That night he had two or three beers in the hotel bar. His friends thought he was drunk as he was very disinhibited and uncharacteristically crude in his language. His speech was rapid and he made a series of lame jokes. When he started dancing on a table he was asked to leave and his teammates took him to his room.

At 3 am, the hotel management were called to his room because of noise disturbance. He had been banging on his teammates' doors dressed in his underwear and inviting them to an all-night party in his room. His speech was very rapid and he couldn't stop laughing. He said he felt on top of the world.

A psychiatrist who was accompanying another team in the same hotel was asked to help and concluded he was probably experiencing an episode of mania. He advised diazepam and olanzapine (10 mg) was also offered. This took a great deal of time and persuasion from the psychiatrist, team manager, and a trusted team-mate. After a second dose of diazepam 4 hours later, he fell asleep and slept for 11 hours. Olanzapine was continued nightly and although he remained a little overfamiliar and restless his more florid symptoms subsided.

He was well enough to travel home 3 days later. He flew with the team doctor and saw a psychiatrist a few days later. Olanzapine was continued for 2 months but stopped because of over-sedation. During this time he was established on treatment with lithium for prophylaxis against further episodes. A contingency plan was developed to prevent and manage sleep disturbance using either melatonin (if competing the next day) or otherwise zopiclone. This was used prophylactically when travelling across time zones. Three years later he has not had a recurrence of either depression or mania.

3.9.3 **Overtraining syndrome**

Assuming no imminent suicide or self-harm risk, then the initial management strategies may focus on addressing training issues. This is done in collaboration with coaching staff. The key is to ensure that exercise intensity is moderated so as to prevent a recurring cycle of OR and OTS. When managing OTS it is necessary to use an objective physiological measure to prevent over-reaching once more. A suggested regimen is a period of complete rest (approximately 2 weeks) then increasing intensity beginning at a relatively low level of intensity (using heart rate as a physiological measure of this, one would be aiming for around 120 bpm) for 20–30 minutes with 1–2 days of complete rest per week and gradually increasing intensity (measured by heart rate) weekly. When an exercise pulse of 160 bpm is reached, the programme can be adjusted to grade the next 6–12 weeks of training, aiming to return to full training by the end of that time. It must be stressed that recovery times are highly variable and regular multidisciplinary evaluation involving coaching and medical staff is needed. Subjective assessment of mood is very sensitive to recovery in OTS and mood ratings can be used as an adjunct to judge how and when to increase the training load.

Other interventions should also be considered. There is an evidence base for psychotherapies in the general population across a range of mental disorders, especially mood disorders, although as yet no sport-specific research. Attention should also be given to adequate sleep, nutrition (especially carbohydrate intake), and to counselling approaches that address ongoing psychosocial stresses. From a mental health perspective, the key issue in OTS is to ensure that significant depressive symptoms are not missed and if present, are adequately assessed and treated.

3.10 **Suicide in sport**

3.10.1 **Prevalence**

Suicide in a high-profile public figure attracts significant media attention and this can distort the perception of suicide prevalence rates. However, there are no reliable statistics on suicide attempts and completed suicide in professional sport; nor indeed any reason to suppose that it is higher or lower than in other groups. Suicide is self-evidently a serious complication of any mental illness and strenuous efforts at prevention alongside good treatment and care are necessary regardless of the prevalence rate. The most important issues in suicide prevention are to be aware that the risk exists and to be able to assess this risk competently. The support of a psychiatrist can be invaluable in these situations.

3.10.2 **Prevention**

Preventative strategies focus on increasing awareness by providing accurate information and education for athletes and professionals in the coaching, medical, and scientific support teams. This is augmented by:

- building the emotional resilience of athletes and teams (see Chapter 9)
- encouraging athletes to be open about their mental well-being and moving away from seeing all symptoms of mental ill health as emotional weakness or frailty
- ensuring high-quality and easily accessible assessment and treatment for any athlete concerned about their mental health.

3.10.3 **Assessment**

There is often reluctance to discuss symptoms of mental health problems within society and within sport. This applies especially in depressive disorders because the sufferer is inclined to evaluate him- or herself in a negative light as a result of the distorted thinking that accompanies depression. This reluctance is especially important when evaluating suicidal thoughts, intentions, and plans.

An enquiry about suicidal thoughts should form part of every psychiatric evaluation and every consultation with a depressed patient. It is a misperception that asking about suicidal thoughts might increase these and make suicide more likely. This is not the case. Indeed, providing an opportunity to frankly discuss feelings can help an individual to identify alternative options to deal with distress and this reduces the risk of suicide. Table 3.1 describes a tool that can facilitate suicide assessment. It is important to note that athletes are often capable of high-level performances in spite of depressive symptoms and even when suicidal thought are present. As an example, in 2009, the German football goalkeeper Robert Enke performed well in an important match just 2 days before he tragically committed suicide.

3.10.4 **Evaluation of the risk of suicide**

Several important features in the thinking and behaviour of those who are contemplating suicide have been described. These can be divided into historical and current risk factors. Historical risk factors include previous suicidal attempts and a family history of suicide.

Table 3.1 Suicide risk assessment tool	

Ask the patient about the following issues *over the last month* (or shorter period for a follow-up assessment):

Questions to explore with individual	If response 'yes' score:
1. Have you had thoughts that you would be better off dead or wish you were dead?	1
2. Have you had thoughts of wanting to harm yourself?	2
3. Have you been thinking of killing yourself/suicide?	6
4. Do you have a suicide plan?	10
5. Have you made any attempt to kill yourself (in the last month or shorter period of time)?	10
6. Have you ever made an attempt to kill yourself?	4

As a rough guide, total the score for the individual:

1–5 points suggests low risk

6–9 points suggests moderate risk

10 or more points suggest high risk.

Source data from *J Clin Psychiatry*, 59(Suppl 20), Sheehan DV *et al.*, The Mini-International Neuropsychiatric Interview (M.I.N.I.): the development and validation of a structured diagnostic psychiatric interview for DSM-IV and ICD-10, p. 22–33, Copyright (1998) Physicians Postgraduate Press, Inc.

3.10.4.1 *Planning*

Perhaps the most important current risk factor for suicide is the presence of active suicidal thoughts, especially when these are associated with planning how to carry out the act. The more detailed the plans the higher the risk, for example, when thoughts include ways of avoiding detection or making arrangements for others after death. An athlete who expresses suicidal thoughts accompanied by a high level of intent to carry out a suicidal act needs rapid assessment, support, and treatment.

3.10.4.2 *Impulsivity*

It is also important to consider levels of impulsivity and factors that might influence this. An individual may not experience suicidal thoughts or plans most of the time. However, if these come into their mind fleetingly and the individual is impulsive, then there is a higher risk they will act on their thoughts. Factors such as alcohol can significantly exacerbate impulsivity.

3.10.4.3 *Emotional constriction*

Emotional and affective constriction has been reported as a risk for suicide. This manifests in verbal and non-verbal communication. The athlete/patient is absorbed by their depressed mood and the content of their conversation is limited and pessimistic in nature. They have a negative appraisal of their capabilities and a depressed perspective on their life ahead. They withdraw from social activities. In sport, this might be misinterpreted as something positive as it could represent psychological preparation and increased concentration prior to performance.

3.10.4.4 *Aggression*

Aggression is normal in many sports and often represents the expression of sporting ambition. However, it is important to be alert to changes in aggressive behaviour. Of special concern are instances when aggression is directed inwardly with self-blame, self-reproach, or even self-injury.

A rating scale for assessment of suicide risk (see Table 3.1) is useful as a starting point but responses need to be interpreted clinically. Other factors that might also increase risk are feelings of hopelessness; psychosocial stresses such as the breakdown of an important relationship; and perceived criticism of the athlete from coaches, club, fans, or the media.

In addition to assessing factors that exacerbate risk it is also vital to explore protective factors. An individual may score highly on the risk assessment tool but in fact be at lower risk. For example, the perceived impact death would have on children and loved ones or certain religious beliefs reduce the likelihood of acting on suicidal thoughts. It is also essential to continuously reassess protective factors since if they start to wane then risk may increase dramatically.

3.10.5 **Management of suicide risk**

The assessment itself is the starting point of any management plan and may decrease risk by instilling hope and identifying immediate supports. Strategies to minimize risk need to be identified alongside protective factors. The initial management plans should make both explicit and identify how risk factors will be reduced and how protective factors will be bolstered. This assessment will highlight risk factors where it is possible to intervene, including treatment of any underlying depressive illness. An assessment must also identify any available support networks. It is easier to manage risk in an athlete who is living at home with a family or partner with whom they have a good relationship than when the athlete is travelling and in a relatively unsupported environment. In general it is better to try to manage the situation with the athlete remaining in their normal environment. Very occasionally, risks will be so high that support networks are unable to ensure that the athlete/patient remains safe. In these instances, admission to an inpatient facility may be needed. Such decisions are difficult and should be made with and by experienced clinicians. Anxiety over the impact of an admission on an individual should not over-ride the need to ensure safety in high-risk situations.

3.11 **Prevention**

We know very little about how to achieve primary prevention in mood disorders. However, it is wise to consider the sport-specific risk factors reviewed in Section 3.4 and where possible to incorporate measures to address these into sports organizations and teams and to have an organizational ethos that supports mental well-being. OTS prevention rests with ensuring that coaching practices and training intensity acknowledge the risk and make sure that training is periodized to allow both over-reaching and rest with super-compensation. Alongside this athletes may need support with lifestyle management and nutrition.

An additional major element of prevention is early detection. Every athlete recognizes symptoms of tiredness, listlessness, and a lack of drive following strenuous training, as well as anxiety related to competition. These symptoms of a possible depressive episode can therefore often be overlooked or misinterpreted as part of a developing OTS, especially if OR and OTS are not seen as specific risk factors for depression. The dilemma for the athlete and their support team is to understand that these symptoms may also be signs of depression and to take appropriate steps for this to be assessed. There is a belief among some that high performances in sport can only be achieved if no clinical significant mental disorder is present. This can lead to symptoms in athletes being ignored or dismissed, with treatment not being given, or athletes being left alone with their symptoms.

There is a need for education across sport to enhance awareness of mood disorders and skills in identifying when expert help is needed. Athletes, coaches, sports physicians, sports psychologists, physiotherapists, and others will benefit from this knowledge. This will require the breakdown of a considerable degree of stigma in many quarters and recognition that depression and other mental disorders are not rare or non-existent in elite performers. The increasing number of psychiatrists with a special interest in high-performance athletes could help to address these problems over time. An interdisciplinary dialogue among all professionals dealing with mental health problems in competitive sport is desirable.

3.11.1 **Secondary prevention**

When an individual athlete has been identified as suffering from a mood disorder then there needs to be a focus on secondary prevention—that is preventing further episodes of illness. With regard to depression, the main evidence is for CBT and continued antidepressant treatment. The general recommendation is for individuals to take antidepressants for 6–12 months after full remission has been achieved and they are free of symptoms. Where there are residual symptoms or a history of multiple episodes the evidence is in favour of longer-term use of antidepressant drugs. It is important to consider this duration of treatment when first starting medication and this highlights the importance of finding medication that is well tolerated.

For bipolar disorder, there are a range of medications that can be taken in the long term to help prevent further episodes of illness. This is a vital part of the management of the illness given its high rate of recurrence. Lithium and quetiapine can be effective in preventing both depressive and manic episodes. Other antipsychotics and valproate tend to be better at preventing episodes of mania than of depression while lamotrigine has the opposite profile.

Both residual symptoms and illness recurrence are common and so secondary prevention in both depression and bipolar disorder can pay enormous dividends.

Further reading

American Psychiatric Association (2013). *Diagnostic and Statistical Manual of Mental Disorders* (5th ed.). Washington, DC: American Psychiatric Association.

Anderson, I.M., Ferrier, I.N., Baldwin, R.C., Cowen, P.J., Howard, L., Lewis, G., et al. (2008). Evidence-based guidelines for treating depressive disorders with antidepressants: a revision of the 2000 British Association for Psychopharmacology guidelines. *J Psychopharmacol* 22(4):343–96. [Available from BAP Consensus Guidelines at http://bap.org.uk/publications.php where updates of this guideline will also be placed.]

Goodwin, G.M. (2009). Evidence-based guidelines for treating bipolar disorder: revised second edition—recommendations from the British Association for Psychopharmacology. *J Psychopharmacol* 23(4):346–88. [Available from BAP Consensus Guidelines at http://bap.org.uk/publications.php where updates of this guideline will also be placed.]

Hirschfeld, R.M., Williams, J.B., Spitzer, R.L., Calabrese, J.R., Flynn, L., Keck, P.E., Jr, et al. Development and validation of a screening instrument for bipolar spectrum disorder: the Mood Disorder Questionnaire. *Am J Psychiatry* 157(11):1873–5.

Meeusen, R., Duclos, M., Foster, C., Fry, A., Gleeson, M., Nieman, D., et al. (2013). Prevention, diagnosis, and treatment of the overtraining syndrome: joint consensus statement of the European College of Sport Science and the American College of Sports Medicine. *Med Sci Sports Exerc* 45(1):186–205.

National Institute for Health and Clinical Excellence (2006). *Bipolar Disorder: The Management of Bipolar Disorder in Adults, Children and Adolescents, in Primary and Secondary Care*. NICE Clinical Guideline 38. London: NICE.

National Institute for Health and Clinical Excellence (2009). *Depression: The Treatment and Management of Depression in Adults (Update)*. NICE Clinical Guideline 91. London: NICE.

Chapter 4

Eating disorders

Alan Currie, Jon Arcelus, and Carolyn Plateau

Key points

- Eating disorders are prevalent across all sports but especially those where weight and/or body shape has a direct impact on performance. These are aesthetic sports (e.g. gymnastics), endurance sports (e.g. distance running), weight category sports (e.g. judo), and antigravity sports (e.g. high jumping).
- Eating disorders negatively impact on athletes' health and performance.
- The sports environment contains additional risk factors for those vulnerable to eating disorders.
- The risks can be managed by adopting appropriate nutritional and coaching practices.
- Although early identification of disorders can be difficult, there are considerable benefits from prompt identification, assessment, and treatment.
- The sports coach can have an important role in the identification and management of eating disorders.
- Recovery and rehabilitation require collaboration between the athlete, his/her support team, and the treating clinical team.

4.1 Introduction

Increasingly refined cross-sectional surveys have established an excess of eating disorder morbidity in sporting populations. Examination and description of the sports environment has helped to explain why sportspeople may be exposed to additional risks. This helps to explain the excess prevalence and informs preventative and risk management strategies. Many large sports organizations have adopted guidelines and/or published position statements on eating disorders. These include the International Olympic Committee, the National Collegiate Athletic Association in the United States, and UK Sport in the United Kingdom.

4.2 **Diagnosis**

In severe cases, the diagnostic label is seldom in doubt but even here migration from one category to another over time is not uncommon. Away from the extremes, the diagnostic separation is less clear and it has become common for some practitioners to think of a spectrum or continuum of eating disorders. The key features of all the categories described in the following sections are summarized in Table 4.1.

4.2.1 **Anorexia nervosa**

This condition is characterized by a restriction of energy intake (relative to requirement) leading to weight loss, which is considered significant for the age, gender, development, and physical health of the individual. In adolescents, this may present as failure to grow as expected rather than as absolute weight loss. Food restriction is accompanied by intense fear of gaining weight or becoming fat, disturbance of self-perception of weight or shape, and lack of recognition of seriously low body weight. In addition, body weight and shape have undue and excessive influence on how the individual evaluates him/herself. It is common to see widespread endocrine disturbance secondary to weight loss and especially in the hypothalamic–pituitary–gonadal (HPG) axis. HPG axis dysfunction leads to amenorrhoea in female sufferers and loss of sexual interest and potency in males but is no longer considered to be part of the diagnostic criteria listed in the Diagnostic and Statistical Manual of Mental Disorders, fifth edition (DSM-5).

4.2.2 **Bulimia nervosa**

In this disorder, overeating binges are frequent (which DSM-5 defines as at least once per week on average, for a minimum of 3 months). Binges involve rapid consumption of large quantities (larger than what most individuals would eat in a similar period of time and under similar circumstances). The individual describes lack of control when consuming these large quantities. Considerable preoccupation with food and food cravings are reported. There is a persistent dread of fatness and a shared characteristic with anorexia nervosa is that self-evaluation is unduly influenced by body shape and weight. Low weight, however, is not a feature of bulimia nervosa. Binges are typically followed by behaviour to counteract the fattening effects of food such as self-induced vomiting, the use of purgatives, fasting, or excessive exercise. Individuals without these compensatory behaviours are diagnosed as suffering from binge-eating disorder.

4.2.3 **Other specified feeding or eating disorders**

A large majority of individuals with abnormal eating behaviours do not meet the full diagnostic criteria for an eating disorder. In these circumstances, the terms 'atypical anorexia/bulimia nervosa' or purging disorder may be used depending on the predominant symptoms. Atypical disorders may not be less serious and features such as extreme purging behaviours may result in considerable harm.

Sport-specific eating disorder syndromes have been described within the field of sport and sports medicine. Although they have not been adopted within the mainstream classification systems, it is important to consider them (see Sections 4.2.4 and 4.2.5).

4.2.4 **Female athlete triad**

The three elements required for this triad are (1) low energy availability, (2) menstrual dysfunction, and (3) low bone mineral density (BMD). Low energy availability occurs either via increased expenditure (training) or reduced intake. As a consequence there will be a HPG axis disruption that will result in osteopenia or osteoporosis (low BMD).

Occasionally, the triad may arise inadvertently and without the presence of the psychological components of an eating disorder such as disturbed body image or morbid dread of fatness. This could occur when a planned increase in training volume is not accompanied by a corresponding adjustment in calorie intake and energy availability either through misunderstanding or ignorance.

4.2.5 **Relative energy deficiency in sport**

Low energy availability (or relative energy deficiency) is both central and primary to the female athlete triad. However, energy deficiency is not exclusive to sportswomen and it is also known that the physiological effects of energy deficiency extend beyond disturbance of menstrual function and compromised bone health. Therefore the term 'female athlete triad' does not fully or accurately describe the condition. Relative energy deficiency in sport (RED-S) has been proposed instead as the preferred term and describes a condition where there is inadequate energy to support the body functions involved in health and performance.

Energy availability is deficient when intake is insufficient to meet the demands of homeostasis, growth, normal daily activities, and exercise. In a sporting context it can be described as the energy that remains to support these physiological functions after exercise/training. It is calculated relative to fat-free mass (FFM) reflecting the higher energy demands to support normal physiology with a larger FFM:

$$\text{Energy availability} (EA) = \frac{\text{energy intake } (EI) - \text{energy expenditure } (EE)}{\text{Fat free mass} (FFM)}$$

An approximate EA value of 45 kcal/kg/day is needed for energy balance in healthy adults and physiological functioning is likely to be significantly compromised at EA values of less than 30 kcal/kg/day.

There are three main routes to low energy availability in sport. It may arise inadvertently, for example, when training load has been increased (higher EE) without a necessary adjustment in dietary intake (EI is unchanged), or it may result from mismanaged or inadequately supervised dietary restrictions (reduced EI). Finally, it may arise out of disordered eating or an eating disorder.

4.2.6 **Disordered eating**

Problematic eating behaviours, unhealthy attitudes to weight and shape, and significant concerns about body image are not only common within the population but have a significant association with the development of eating disorders. Unless a clinical syndrome is present, these attitudes, behaviours, and concerns are usually described in the broad term 'disordered eating'. Common examples of disordered eating could include fasting and other types of food restriction such as skipping meals, extreme faddy diets, the non-therapeutic use of diet pills, diuretics and enemas, vomiting and other forms of purging, and excessive exercise. Disordered eating is frequently co-morbid with other psychiatric conditions such as depression.

4.2.7 **Athletic eating**

Sportspeople striving for excellence will do out-of-the-ordinary things such as training to near exhaustion repeatedly. An athlete may also pay meticulous attention to his or her diet (because it fuels performance) and to his or her weight (because excess will hinder performance). This may bear a resemblance to the thinking and behaviour of the eating disorder sufferer. In the healthy athlete, these attitudes and behaviours are directed towards enhancing sporting achievement, not an end in themselves, an activity undertaken compulsively nor with weight loss as the primary objective. Associated features that would raise concern about the presence of an eating disorder are fear of fatness, self-evaluation unduly influenced by body shape or weight, and significant physiological disturbance secondary to energy deficiency.

Table 4.1 Eating disorder spectrum in sport

Anorexia nervosa	Bulimia nervosa	Female athlete triad (FAT)	Relative energy deficiency in sport (RED-S)	Disordered eating	Athletic eating
Food/energy restriction Weight loss or growth delay Self-evaluation by weight/shape Fear of weight gain Distorted perception of weight shape Secondary endocrine disturbance[a]	Frequent food binges with loss of control Compensatory behaviours (e.g. vomiting, purging, exercise) Self-evaluation by weight/shape Food craving and preoccupation	Low energy availability (EA) Menstrual dysfunction Low bone mineral density	Low energy availability (EA <30 kcal/kg/day) Widespread physiological disturbance May be secondary to increased training, inadequate diet or disordered eating/eating disorder	Problematic but subclinical disturbances of: Eating attitudes and behaviours (e.g. missed meals, diet pills, purges, excessive exercise) Body image	Detailed attention to diet Weight concerns Both motivated primarily by athletic performance
Atypical if not all criteria present	Atypical if not all criteria present			Strongly predictive of future eating disorder	Disordered eating attitudes and behaviours not present
	Binge eating disorder (BED) if no compensatory behaviours				

[a] Not part of DSM-5 criteria.

4.3 **Prevalence**

Estimating the prevalence of eating disorders in sport can be problematic. Examining heterogeneous populations (from many sports and/or across a wide range of abilities and level of participation) may fail to detect pockets of high prevalence in high-risk sports. Using screening instruments that are not validated for sporting populations can produce both over- and underestimated prevalence rates. Screening tests may overestimate prevalence by ascribing pathology or caseness to 'athletic eating' because of its similarity to the thinking and behaviour found in eating disorders. Alternatively, the need for athletes to keep their problems secret or risk sanctions can result in underestimation.

Whilst it is usual to think primarily of weight loss when considering eating disorders, the commonest disorders are bulimic in nature where weight is frequently within the normal range. In sport, an emphasis on weight can be especially unhelpful and objective measures of weight are unreliable indicators of eating disorders for two important reasons.

Firstly, body mass index (BMI) is not necessarily an indicator of abnormality in sports that attract individuals with an unusually lean body composition. There is a risk of incorrectly identifying a disorder in those who are simply constitutionally unusual and at, or just beyond, the extremes of normal.

Secondly, in many power and strength sports there will be very muscular individuals with an unusually high body weight or BMI. Individuals with this body type may need to lose a great deal of weight to 'qualify' for a diagnosis according to strict eating disorder criteria. This can mask the descent into an eating disorder even in the presence of other clear eating disorder signs and symptoms.

Issues of misestimation of prevalence were addressed in the large 2004 study by Sundgot-Borgen and Torstveit (see Table 4.2). Subjects were a homogeneous group of elite performers large enough to include significant numbers in each sport studied. Screening questionnaires were supplemented by detailed clinical interviews and the study also included male subjects and a control population.

The overall prevalence of eating disorders in female athletes was found to be 20% in the elite sports group and 9% in the control group; 8% of males in elite sports were identified as having an eating disorder, which represents a 16-fold increase compared to the control group prevalence of 0.5%. This suggests that the sports environment may make a proportionally larger contribution to risk for sportsmen than for sportswomen. Several sports emerge with especially high prevalence rates. For females, these are aesthetic, weight category, and endurance sports and for males, antigravity, weight category, and endurance sports (Figure 4.1).

4.4 **Aetiological factors**

Eating disorders are usually seen as having multifactorial origins with complex interactions between environmental, biological, psychological, and genetic factors and personality traits. Some factors, such as personality, are considered to be vulnerability factors, predisposing to the development of disorders whilst others can precipitate or maintain the condition.

Table 4.2 Eating disorder (ED) prevalence by sports type (males and females)

Sports	Examples	Female		Male	
		ED rate	%	ED rate	%
Aesthetic	Gymnastics, diving	22/52	42	0/13	0
Weight class	Judo, wrestling	16/53	30	14/79	18
Endurance	Running, orienteering	24/104	24	14/149	9
Technical	Golf	12/72	17	4/97	4
Ball game	Football, handball	39/252	16	14/277	5
Antigravitation	High-jump, ski jumping	1/10	< 1	8/37	22
Power	Sprints, weight-lifting	1/31	< 1	1/18	< 1
Motor	Karting	0/0	–	0/17	0
Total		115/572	20	55/687	8
Controls		52/574	9	3/629	< 1

Adapted from *Clin. J. Sports Med.*, 14, Sundgot-Borgen, J and Torstveit MK, Prevalence of eating disorders in elite athletes is higher than in the general population, p. 24–32, Copyright (2004), with permission from Wolters Kluwer Health, Inc.

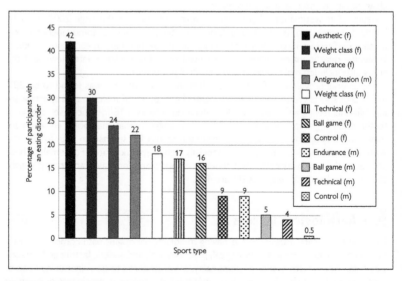

Figure 4.1 Prevalence by type of sport.

Source data from *Clinical Journal of Sport Medicine*, 14(1), Sundgot-Borgen, J and Torstveit MK, Prevalence of eating disorders in elite athletes is higher than in the general population, p. 24–32, Copyright (2004) Wolters Kluwer Health.

Athletes are vulnerable to eating disorders for the same reasons as anyone else and sport in isolation does not 'cause' eating disorders. However, there are sport-specific factors that have been shown, for example, to precipitate and maintain body dissatisfaction known to be a risk for an eating disorder. Awareness of the many aetiological factors in sport is helpful in understanding the excess prevalence found in sport. Collectively, knowledge of these factors will inform the preventative and risk management strategies that are necessary within sport. The following section will discuss in detail the sport-related aetiological factors that have been linked to eating disorders.

4.4.1 Vulnerability factors

Personality traits—many personality traits that are functional for the aspiring athlete (functional in the sense that they are associated with achievement and success) bear a similarity to attributes found in the eating disorders sufferer. These include perfectionism, mental toughness, and commitment (to training/exercise). Perfectionism can include both high standard-setting and critical self-evaluation. Setting high standards does not appear to be associated with negative outcomes but when accompanied by excessive self-criticism can be problematic.

Compulsive and excessive exercise—exercise can help mood regulation. An unhealthy relationship with exercise can develop when this is the only way of coping with stress. Mood regulation can become the primary aim of exercise and the individual becomes anxious if unable to exercise. Exercise is not enjoyable, becomes a chore, and can be said to be compulsive. In addition, if exercise is curtailed (e.g. by injury), the athlete is not only stressed and anxious but has had the primary means of dealing with this removed. In these circumstances, a lack of other coping skills can lead to more unhealthy attempts to regain a degree of control, such as dietary restrictions.

'Excessive' exercise is a qualitative rather than a quantitative evaluation and is best determined by the motivation that drives exercise rather than volume or intensity. For example, exercise with a primary purpose of weight control, exercise undertaken compulsively (perhaps even in secret), or an unhealthy dependence on exercise to regulate mood may be features of excessive exercise even when the absolute volume of exercise is relatively modest.

Aesthetics—in some sports the judgement of performance is associated with a particular and desirable body shape. These aesthetic evaluations will promote that body composition in competitors.

Competitive thinness—sporting achievement is driven by a competitive desire and this can generalize to a drive to be not just faster/higher/stronger but also leaner. Developing athletes may strive for the body weight of those they desire to emulate.

Early sport-specific training—increases vulnerability perhaps because younger athletes in an early stage of their sporting development may select a sport less suited to their eventual body type or because early specialization is associated with competing at a higher competitive level than is appropriate for their stage of psychological maturation.

Sport as an identity—if an athlete's life is filled only with sport and lacking other activities then their sense of identity is so closely linked to sports participation that any event threatening this identity will have a significant impact on self-esteem. Injury, retirement, or not being selected for competition is then a more significant loss. A loss such as this removes many key features of the athlete's identity including a sense of achievement, their most significant role in life, a sense of belonging, and a way of dealing with stress and controlling weight. An eating disorder can substitute for some aspects of this lost identity.

4.4.2 **Precipitating and maintaining factors**

Making weight—this is a necessity in weight category sports such as judo, boxing, or Olympic wrestling and failure to make weight will lead to exclusion. This can promote rapid and extreme weight-loss measures similar to those seen in bulimia nervosa. In some sports, these measures are seen as almost a cultural norm and present from a young age.

Dieting—weight loss is especially risky if unsupervised, rapid, and without a clear target or end point. Most athletes who have suffered from an eating disorder report that a period of dieting preceded the onset of the condition.

Body weight and performance—body weight is closely linked to endurance performance and weight loss may still be associated with a temporary improvement in performance even if the athlete is already very lean.

Sports clothing—revealing attire is an additional risk factor especially in an environment of competitive thinness and aesthetic evaluations. This is compounded when critical self-evaluation (one feature of perfectionism) is also present.

Negative life events—athletes are especially vulnerable to the negative life events that result in loss of their sporting identity. These will include events such as retirement or injuries which interrupt training and competition. When the sporting identity is threatened, this impacts in a number of ways to increase the risk of developing an eating disorder (see Section 4.4.1).

The body as an object/machine—the pursuit of excellence may lead an athlete to become preoccupied by physiological parameters and their measurement (and often these are measured by sophisticated technological means). The athlete can then come to see his/her body as an object which is detached from his/her internal experiences. This problem is magnified if the body/object is seen as imperfect and in need of modification.

Critical or derogatory comments—about shape, weight, and body composition from peers, family members, or a coach have been found to be associated with the development of an eating disorder. This is especially the case when critical self-evaluations are also a feature of the athlete's psychopathology.

Organizational culture—in some sports, pathological weight control measures are encouraged and reinforced. In addition there are many sports where it can be hard to access psychiatric expertise and where there is considerable stigma attached to showing apparent psychological 'frailty'.

Timely access to treatment—denial is prominent in many eating disorders and may delay presentation. In addition, many athletes have lifestyles that make it harder to access mainstream healthcare and are subject to stigma when disclosing psychological problems. Delays in assessment may allow a problem to become entrenched and delays in treatment may lead to physical complications that are harder to reverse.

4.5 **Prevention**

Having an eating disorder such as anorexia nervosa is associated with significant morbidity and mortality. The seriousness of these conditions once established is a powerful argument for extensive efforts at prevention.

Coaches and other members of the support team need information on the health risks of restricted eating and the importance of ensuring adequate energy availability especially in athletes who are still growing. If it is necessary to set a weight-loss objective with an athlete then this should be done by medical and nutritionally qualified staff rather than a coach, and not in an athlete who is still growing. Strict policies may be necessary in sports where unhealthy weight-loss strategies are common, for example, in some weight category sports. Critical or derogatory comments about shape, weight, and body composition may also require policing and public weighing should be actively discouraged.

The arguments for developing preventative practices can be extended to the need for screening and early detection. There are essentially two approaches to screening. The first is to educate those who work with athletes on the likely presenting symptoms of eating disorders and how to distinguish these from normal 'athletic' concerns about shape and weight (see Section 4.2.7). Early detection means not only knowing what to look for but also looking hard and often. Special attention should be given to those athletes from 'at-risk' groups (due to their type of sport and personality factors) and to injured athletes.

The second approach (and they are by no means mutually exclusive) is to introduce formal screening instruments into regular medical examinations. For example, a preseason medical could include the five-item SCOFF questionnaire (Table 4.3) as part of general health assessment. The SCOFF questionnaire has a reported sensitivity of 85% and specificity of 90% in primary care settings. It is a screening instrument that raises suspicion about a possible disorder and is not a diagnostic tool. However, self-completed questionnaires of this type have not been specifically developed for athletes and depend on athletes giving honest answers. This may be hard to rely on as individuals with eating disorders frequently show high levels of ambivalence and athletes may fear the consequences of disclosing eating disorders symptoms.

Table 4.3 SCOFF questionnaire				
1. Do you make yourself **S**ick because you feel uncomfortably full?	Yes	☐	No	☐
2. Do you worry you have lost **C**ontrol over how much you eat?	Yes	☐	No	☐
3. Have you lost more than **O**ne stone (7Kgs/14lbs) in a three month period?	Yes	☐	No	☐
4. Do you believe yourself to be **F**at when others say you are too thin?	Yes	☐	No	☐
5. Would you say that **F**ood dominates your life?	Yes	☐	No	☐

A score of 2 or more indicates the need for a more detailed assessment.

Reproduced from *The BMJ*, 319, Morgan, J. *et al*, The SCOFF questionnaire: assessment of a new screening tool for eating disorders, Copyright (1999), with permission from BMJ Publishing Group Ltd.

A high index of suspicion is recommended and it is especially important to be vigilant with adolescent female athletes where 90% of peak bone mass is attained by the age of 18. Energy deficiency in the mid-teenage years will have long-term consequences for health and for sustaining a sporting career into adulthood.

When one element of disorder is present (e.g. menstrual irregularity, weight loss, or failure to grow), this should prompt inquiry and further exploration. Deteriorating performances, recurrent illness, and recurrent or non-healing injuries may also be warning signs of energy deficiency and a sustained catabolic state. Mood changes and especially symptoms of low mood and irritability can also be early signs.

4.6 **Assessment, treatment, and recovery**

As with eating disorders in other contexts, considerable resistance or at best ambivalence is common and this complicates and delays the assessment process. The first step towards recovery is motivating the individual to accept help and to make changes. About one-third of athletes with eating disorders voluntarily disclose their disorder while approximately two-thirds are approached by others in the first instance. Athletes who disclose usually do so to their teammates or coach. When disclosure is initiated by others, the experience is often reported in a negative light by the athlete.

4.6.1 **Motivation and readiness to accept help**

Members of the support team may often find themselves in a position to motivate an athlete to accept help and support. For this reason, coaches and others in the athlete's support team need to understand the process of disclosure and motivation for change.

The first step is to discuss any concerns openly with the athlete. Good advice is to make an approach directly, early, supportively, and confidentially. Directness is a sign of honesty and will reduce the risk of unhelpful collusion with any secrecy and denial on the part of the athlete. An early approach is necessary to prevent further deterioration in physical health, mental health, and performance. An ambivalent athlete will need support and encouragement to make the step to further assessment and possible treatment and a critical or blaming attitude may exaggerate the athlete's resistance. Confidentiality in respect of other team members must be respected as in all other medical matters.

This first discussion can be used to assess the stage of the athlete's readiness to change. Several stages of motivation for change have been described (Figure 4.2).

Those who are close to individuals such as parents, partners, or coaches can help the move from one stage to the next. If a person is not in the 'action stage', talking to them about change may not be helpful. It may be more fruitful at that point to take an approach of weighing up the pros and cons of change. Pushing someone to change before they have the opportunity to contemplate this and develop determination may generate resistance and move them back to a less motivated stage.

4.6.2 **Contracts**

Contracts are by definition two-way agreements and they allow all parties to be explicit in advance about what will be offered and what will be expected in return. The contract of a professional athlete can be used to describe what medical support

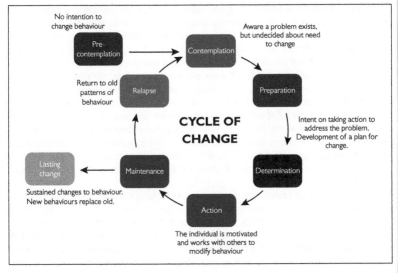

Figure 4.2 Stages of motivation for change.

Source data from *Journal of Consulting and Clinical Psychology*, 5, Prochaska, J. and DiClemente, C., Stages and processes of self-change in smoking: toward an integrative model of change, p. 390–395, Copyright (1983) American Psychological Association.

will be provided, in what circumstances, and how the athlete would be expected to use this support—for example, being expected to participate in screening and to take advantage of assessment and treatment when offered. Contracts may also explicitly state the criteria to judge an athlete's fitness to train or compete. However, this is often not absolute and requires clinical judgement in the athlete's best interests (see Section 4.6.4). Finally, contracts can describe the circumstances that will lead to exclusion or contract termination—usually deteriorating performances, whether or not the result of ill health or injury. Athletes, coaches, and sports organizations should expect contracts to apply the same principles for both physical and mental disorders.

These elements of a contract can also form the basis of the more informal relationship that exists between an athlete competing at a lower or more recreational level and his/her coach.

4.6.3 **Access to assessment**

When an eating disorder is diagnosed and an athlete is motivated to get help it is important to be clear about how further assessment and treatment will be accessed. Both a medical and psychiatric evaluation will be necessary. Professional athletes with an extensive support team may have ready access to this kind of evaluation (although in most areas a 'team psychiatrist' is a rarity), others will need to know how to make best use of whatever healthcare system is available to them. Access to assessment and treatment for injuries and physical complaints may be funded by sports bodies but in many cases equivalent mental health expertise is less readily available.

Primary care medical services (e.g. the team doctor or athlete's general practitioner) can have an important role in beginning the medical evaluation (see Box 4.1). In cases of RED-S that have arisen inadvertently through failure to match energy requirements to training load, dietary advice and nutritional support may be the only interventions needed. In milder and subclinical conditions, sound nutritional advice and psychological support may be sufficient to effect the necessary changes. A monitoring arrangement is needed in these cases to ensure that problems are genuinely resolving.

In most other circumstances more specialist help will be required. There can be difficulties accessing specialist eating disorders services and long waiting lists are a common complaint of athletes. Many specialist services have strict entry criteria such a low BMI of 15 or are 'anorexia nervosa only' services. When a disorder is so closely linked to ambivalence then difficulties in accessing services can collude with the patient's stance and reinforce the belief that there is nothing wrong or that there is only a minor problem.

In high-risk or high-prevalence sports it can be helpful to be clear in advance about the pathway to assessment and treatment. This can be done, for example, by forming links with local treatment centres, supporting athletes to consult their personal doctor, and having explicit referral criteria and pathways. Clear policies and pathways will help to remove anxieties from sport bodies, coaches, sports medicine staff, and other members of the support team, as well as to encourage early intervention when an eating problem is suspected.

4.6.4 **Medical evaluation**

The initial medical evaluation will provide the information that may help to decide about the safety of continued participation or to inform the modifications of training/exercise that will be necessary. The medical evaluation should be undertaken by a physician who has experience in the field. Occasionally a sufficiently experienced eating disorders psychiatrist may feel able to undertake the medical evaluation.

Bone scans are usually interpreted with reference to population normative data for age and sex. Athletes in weight-bearing sports will have BMD that is on average 5–15% greater than non-athletes. This influences the interpretation of bone scan data and a BMD Z score of between −1.0 and −2.0 should be considered abnormal in such an

---

Box 4.1 The initial medical evaluation

- Full blood count
- Urea and electrolytes
- Magnesium, phosphate, zinc, and ionized calcium
- Glucose
- Liver function tests
- Thyroid function tests
- Oestrogen, progesterone, luteinizing hormone and follicle-stimulating hormone (in bulimia only if menstrual irregularity)
- ECG
- Dual-energy X-ray absorptiometry (DXA) bone scan if amenorrhoea of more than 1 year.

athlete. In non-athletic populations, only Z scores of less than −2.0 are considered to represent significant lowering of BMD (osteoporosis).

The results of the initial medical evaluation will be the primary determinants in deciding how much or how little participation is advisable. It is regrettably rare for this to be a simple decision and there is no single measure that can guide. The medical evaluation determines health status which is used to evaluate participation risk but this risk is in turn modified by factors specific to the sporting environment.

At one end of the spectrum there will be serious medical complications of energy deficiency that are absolute contraindications to any exercise participation and at the other end of the spectrum the results will provide sufficient reassurance to allow the training and competitive programme to continue unaltered. Most athletes will lie somewhere between extremes. In these circumstances, the training and competition programme can be modified to take account of medical complications, to help restore energy balance, and to promote recovery.

Absolute contraindications include serious electrolyte imbalance, severe musculoskeletal injury, and haemodynamic instability. The athlete would only be cleared to resume training when the relevant physical parameters had stabilized. If the outcome of the medical examination is a situation of low risk with appropriate energy availability, normal hormonal and metabolic function, and healthy BMD and musculoskeletal system then few if any modifications will be needed.

For most athletes the decision on how much participation to permit will need a judgement on the severity and importance of several factors. These include abnormal but not acutely dangerous physiological profile (e.g. hormonal abnormalities), energy balance, weight loss/restricted growth, and BMD. Progression is a second important consideration. The initial aim of modifications to training or exercise is to arrest any deterioration and begin the process of physical rehabilitation. If parameters are worsening or failing to progress then more stringent modifications may be needed. Lack of progression in psychological therapy may be another consideration.

Finally, the sports environment itself will act as an important 'decision modifier'. If the athlete is in the off-season then perhaps rest can be more readily advised to restore energy balance; musculoskeletal considerations may need more emphasis in contact and impact sports, and there may be a very psychologically unhealthy team environment that would merit more prolonged non-participation.

In all cases it is the medical rather than the coaching team that should drive participation decisions. In this way conflicts of interest between athlete and coach can be avoided. In any case, the risks are in large part the result of medical complications necessitating medically led decision-making.

4.6.5 **Psychiatric evaluation**

A psychiatric assessment will not only confirm the diagnosis through careful history taking and examination of the athlete's mental state but will formulate the problem in terms of underlying vulnerability, relevant triggers, and maintenance factors. This requires the same competencies as any other psychiatric diagnostic formulation. The assessment consultation begins with a willingness to engage the individual by understanding the context in which they have become ill and includes consideration of additional 'sport-specific' risk factors in predisposition, precipitating, and perpetuating factors.

The athlete's predisposing vulnerability will need to be explored including factors such as perfectionism especially where this coincides with low self-esteem and critical or negative self-evaluation. Important triggers for disordered eating include critical comments and evaluations from significant others, life events (and in a sporting context even minor injuries can be major events), and life changes such as leaving home or relationship difficulties. As well as exploring the athlete's internal world, questions should also be asked about the athlete's external environment and in particular attitude to weight, eating, dieting, and body shape within that environment.

It is important to take an adequate exercise history. Clinicians should understand the athlete's current attitude to exercise. In particular they should note any recent shifts in attitudes and behaviours from training that is directed by a performance programme and motivated by achieving sporting goals, towards compulsive, additional, or secretive exercise. The use of exercise as the primary means of controlling unpleasant mood states such as anxiety and depression should raise particular concern. The chronology of the athlete's exercising behaviour is also important. This will include determining the onset of excessive exercise as this may predate the onset of disordered eating. Other factors to consider are the impact of puberty on performance, evidence of a performance decrement (or a plateau in attainment), and if the athlete has found him/herself at an early age competing at too high a level for his/her emotional maturity.

The psychiatric evaluation will also clarify and quantify psychiatric risk factors and protective factors. Psychiatric risk includes the risk of suicide and self-harm and the possibility of co-morbid conditions such as depression, anxiety disorders, obsessive–compulsive disorder, and substance misuse.

4.7 Treatment

Psychotherapy, in one of its many forms, is the mainstay of eating disorders treatment with medication usually reserved for the treatment of comorbid conditions. The major difficulty when working with an individual with an eating disorder is that treatment requires active participation in psychotherapy. Attending appointments is not enough.

In anorexia nervosa, there is a growing evidence base for a range of psychotherapeutic approaches including cognitive behavioural therapy (CBT), cognitive analytical therapy (CAT), psychodynamically informed therapy, and interpersonal psychotherapy (IPT). In CBT, the patient is supported to challenge and rebuild maladaptive thinking and behaviour. A modified form of CBT specifically for use in eating disorders (CBT-E) has been developed and focuses on core problems of perfectionism, low self-esteem, managing interpersonal problems, and difficulties coping with unpleasant mood states. Psychodynamic approaches recognize that early experiences and in some cases family dynamics can contribute to eating disorder psychopathology. These approaches support the patient to attend to unpleasant early experiences and to resolve psychological conflicts. Family-based therapy is the treatment of choice for adolescents and actively involves parents/carers in treatment. IPT seems particularly effective when bingeing and compensatory behaviours such as purging are prominent.

Therapy is usually weekly and for 20–40 weeks depending on diagnosis, severity, and the mode of therapy. Research has demonstrated that bulimic-like disorders, such as bulimia nervosa or binge eating disorders, respond to 20 sessions of CBT or

16–20 sessions of IPT and both therapies are recommended in UK national guidelines. The treatment of anorexia nervosa is more complex and currently there is limited evidence on the most effective treatment. Many clinical services offer 40 sessions of CBT-E. Psychodynamic therapy is also used in many clinical services for the treatment of anorexia nervosa and anorexia nervosa-like disorders and usually for about 1 year of weekly sessions.

For mild disorders a graded approach of offering self-help and guided self-help may be useful.

Therapy should be delivered by a suitably trained and qualified therapist or therapy team. Experience of sport can be helpful but is not essential. An ability to understand the context in which an individual has become ill (in this case sport) is common to all therapies and is a mandatory competency for any therapist.

Recent research has identified that the involvement of the coach in the treatment can aid recovery and progress back to sports activities. A sports coach can bring helpful insights into the formulation of the disorder. Furthermore, his/her collaboration will be necessary in managing any restrictions on exercise and in supporting a gradual resumption of sports activities on recovery.

Medication should be used cautiously as cardiac side effects are reported for many psychotropic drugs. This is especially important in those who may have other cardiac vulnerability (e.g. via electrolyte and especially potassium disturbance) and are continuing to exercise. Selective serotonin reuptake inhibiting antidepressants such as fluoxetine can help reduce the frequency of binge episodes and low-dose antipsychotic medications may help reduce anxiety and compulsive behaviours in anorexia nervosa. Otherwise medication is primarily used in the treatment of comorbid conditions such as depressive and anxiety disorders and obsessive–compulsive disorder.

4.8 **Recovery**

There are four major sport-specific considerations that come into play as the athlete/patient progresses from assessment through treatment to recovery and each requires collaboration between the clinical world and the world of sport.

The first consideration is medical stability. Is there a medical contraindication to training/competition such as an electrolyte imbalance, electrocardiogram (ECG) abnormality, or stress fracture? Are these medical concerns of a severity and urgency that immediate action is necessary? These considerations are essentially the same as those which may have led to restrictions on training and competing following the initial medical evaluation.

If there is no immediate medical contraindication to continuing or resuming exercise then the second consideration is the athlete's nutritional status and the key question is whether or not calorie intake is adequate to meet the demands of exercise (see Section 4.2.5).

If nutrition and energy availability are sufficient then a graded return to exercise may be considered although this will be dependent on the third consideration—an observed reduction in disordered eating behaviours and progress in therapy. Progress in therapy is then rewarded by resumption of activity that acts as an incentive for further progress in therapy, creating a virtuous spiral.

The fourth aspect to consider is the risk that returning to training and competition will exacerbate the illness. In many cases, a return to training and competition will be viewed positively. For others, the sports arena may prove sufficiently toxic for the condition to resurface, necessitating a review of the process of return. This will include reviewing the nature and timing of return—was it too early, was progress in therapy overestimated, was there sufficient attention to modifying the relevant risk factors for that athlete? For a few, returning to a lower competitive level or even an exit strategy will be the best option. Clearly at each stage a high level of collaboration between the coach/support team and the clinical team is necessary and should always have the athlete/patient at the centre of any decision and consenting to information being shared.

Further reading

American College of Sports Medicine (2007). The female athlete triad. Position stand. *Med Sci Sports Exerc* 39(10):1867–82.

American Psychiatric Association (2013). *Diagnostic and Statistical Manual of Mental Disorders* (5th ed.). Washington, DC: American Psychiatric Association.

Beals, KA. (2004). *Disordered Eating Amongst Athletes: A Comprehensive Guide for Health Professionals*. Champaign, IL: Human Kinetics.

Currie, A. and Crosland, J. (2009). Responding to eating disorders in sport—UK guidelines. *Nutr Food Sci* 39(6):619–26.

Currie, A. and Morse, ED. (2005). Eating disorders in athletes: managing the risks. *Clin Sports Med* 24:871–3.

Dosil, J. (2008). *Eating Disorders in Athletes*. Chichester: Wiley.

Morgan, J.F., Reid, F., and Lacey, J.H. (1999). The SCOFF questionnaire: assessment of a new screening tool for eating disorders. *BMJ* 319:1467–8.

Mountjoy, M., Sundgot-Borgen, J., Burke, L., Carter, S., Constantini, N., LeBrun, C., *et al.* (2014). The IOC consensus statement: beyond the female athlete triad—relative energy deficiency in sport (RED-S). *Br J Sports Med* 48:491–7.

National Institute for Health and Clinical Excellence (2004). *Eating Disorders: Core Interventions in the Treatment and Management of Anorexia Nervosa, Bulimia Nervosa and Related Eating Disorders*. Clinical Guideline 9. London: NICE. [Available from: https://www.nice.org.uk/guidance/cg9]

Plateau, C.R., McDermott, H.J., Arcelus, J., and Meyer, C. (2014). Identifying and preventing disordered eating among athletes: perceptions of track and field coaches. *Psychol Sport Exerc* 15(6):721–8.

Prochaska, J. and DiClemente, C. (1983). Stages and processes of self-change in smoking: toward an integrative model of change. *J Consult Clin Psychol* 5:390–5.

Schmidt, U. and Treasure, J. (1996). *Getting Better Bit(e) by Bit(e)*. Hove: Psychology Press.

Sundgot-Borgen, J. and Torstveit, M.K. (2004). Prevalence of eating disorders in elite athletes is higher than in the general population. *Clin J Sport Med* 14:25–32.

Thompson, R.A. and Sherman, R.T. (2010). *Eating Disorders in Sport*. New York: Routledge.

UK Sport (2007). *Eating Disorders in Sport: A Guideline Framework for Practitioners Working with High Performance Sportsmen and Women*. [Available from: http://www.uksport.gov.uk/publications/]

Chapter 5

Substance misuse

Pamela Walters, Andrea Hearn, and Alan Currie

Key points

- Substances that are commonly misused in the general population are also misused in sport. In addition, many athletes misuse performance-enhancing drugs.

- Psychiatric expertise is helpful in evaluating and understanding both of these problems and increases the likelihood of being able to offer appropriate interventions.

- Education and awareness will promote more effective screening and early detection of problems. This increases the likelihood of interventions being offered and of those interventions being effective.

- The athlete's stage of change is crucial in being able to offer effective treatment and may itself be amenable to intervention. Sportspeople are motivated individuals and are therefore well placed to engage with and benefit from treatment.

5.1 Introduction

Substances have been used throughout human history. Misuse is defined as the non-therapeutic use of a drug in a manner that is potentially harmful. Similarly, in sport the use of substances with the intention of enhancing performance is likely as old as sport itself and defined as the use or misuse of a prohibited substance—a substance that is unethical and unfair in a sporting context and may also be harmful. The term 'doping' is southern African in origin and derived from a primitive alcoholic drink used as a stimulant prior to a ceremonial dance. The term is now commonly used to describe the use of performance-enhancing drugs (PEDs) in the sporting arena.

Early recorded use of drugs in major sporting events includes strychnine by the winner of the 1904 Olympic marathon. Later, in the 1960 Rome Olympics, a cyclist died having taken a stimulant. By 1967, the International Olympics Committee had banned the use of PEDs in competition and compulsory doping controls were instituted shortly thereafter. Drug testing was initially restricted to competitions but in recent years out-of-competition and random testing has been advocated and implemented as a more powerful deterrent and more likely to yield positive results.

The use of substances occurs across a continuum of acceptability. Some drugs (e.g. caffeine) are taken routinely, culturally accepted, and perhaps even viewed in a positive light. Even when use is legal and routine, approaches may vary. For example, some cultures prohibit alcohol, some restrict its use through high taxation or other selling restrictions, and in others it is freely available. Others substances, which may be widely used, are socially and culturally accepted despite knowledge of their potential to have harmful effects (e.g. nicotine). Some substances are used as therapeutic medication either available for all to buy (over the counter (OTC)) or when sanctioned by a suitably qualified healthcare professional (a prescription). Some prescriptions will be for drugs that would otherwise be prohibited and open to misuse (e.g. benzodiazepines and some opiates). Finally, some substances are prohibited and only available illicitly.

Within competitive sport there is a similar continuum (Figure 5.1). Many substances are accepted and used routinely to enhance performance. This includes nutritional supplements, hydration aids, and energy drinks. Some drugs (e.g. caffeine) are allowed provided they are not used in great excess and an arbitrary upper limit is defined. Others may be allowed within the rules to treat common ailments either as OTC medications or when approved by a licensed medical practitioner (in which case a Therapeutic Use Exemption (TUE) may be needed). Importantly in these instances medication is for the treatment of a health condition that would otherwise impair performance. It is sanctioned as it restores health and contributes to the 'level playing field'. Prohibited substances and methods unfairly and artificially enhance performance whether or not they are harmful (although many are). Within this category are those that are banned only in some sports or only during competition (e.g. in some sports, alcohol or beta blockers) and those that are prohibited at all times (e.g. in most sports, anabolic steroids).

Since 1999, the World Anti-Doping Agency (WADA) has assumed overall responsibility for policy, research, and for overseeing drug testing programmes. It publishes the World Anti-Doping Code, which lists the substances, and methods that are prohibited in and out of competition (http://www.wada-ama.org/) and the list is reviewed annually.

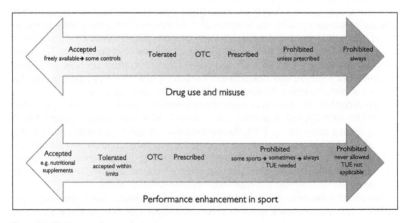

Figure 5.1 Continuum of use and misuse.

5.2 **Classification**

Classificatory systems in common usage share an approach of classifying misuse both by type of drug and by degree of harm.

Types of drug specified in the 10th version of the International Classification of Diseases (ICD-10) are:

- alcohol
- opioids
- cannabinoids
- sedative hypnotics
- cocaine and other stimulants
- hallucinogens
- tobacco
- volatile solvents.

Multiple substance misuse and misuse of other (or unspecified) substances are also classified. This classification system also recognizes pathological gambling and use of non-dependent drugs.

It is also important to consider the impact of the substance used and to separate acute intoxication from longer-term problems. ICD-10 describes harmful use and dependence; the Diagnostic and Statistical Manual of Mental Disorders, fifth edition (DSM-5) classifies the degree of harm as mild, moderate, or severe according to the number of associated symptoms and problems that are seen. A list of 11 symptoms is described:

1. Taken in larger amounts or over a longer period than was intended.
2. Persistent desire or unsuccessful efforts to cut down or control use.
3. A great deal of time is spent in activities necessary to obtain the substance, use it, or recover from its effects.
4. Craving, or a strong desire or urge to use.
5. Failure to fulfil major role obligations at work, school, or home.
6. Continued use despite persistent or recurrent social or interpersonal problems.
7. Important social, occupational, or recreational activities are given up or reduced.
8. Recurrent use in situations in which it is physically hazardous.
9. Continued use despite knowledge of a persistent or recurrent physical or psychological problem that is likely to have been caused or exacerbated by the substance.
10. Tolerance, as defined by either of the following:
    - A need for markedly increased amounts to achieve intoxication or desired effect
    - A markedly diminished effect with the same amount of the substance.
11. Withdrawal, as manifest by either of the following:
    - The characteristic withdrawal syndrome for that substance
    - Substance (or closely related substance) is taken to relieve or avoid withdrawal symptoms.

Where only two or three symptoms are seen, the misuse is defined as mildly harmful. If there are four or five symptoms this is defined as moderately harmful use and when there are six or more symptoms this is categorized as severe harm. For gambling disorder, the criteria are slightly different; four or five symptoms = mild, six or seven = moderate, and eight or more = severe.

5.3 **Classification within sports**

It is helpful to classify the misuse of PEDs in a similar manner, firstly by the type of drug being used and secondly by the nature of that use (for full details see http://list.wada-ama.org). PEDs may be banned at all times, only during competition, only in certain sports, or only above certain limits, and may be allowed if they are needed to treat a medical condition (see Figure 5.1). The list is continually updated.

In sport, there are seven broad classes of drug that may be misused to enhance performance and that are prohibited in at least some sports, some of the time:

- Drugs that increase muscle mass and strength (e.g. anabolic steroids)
- Drugs that increase oxygen carrying capacity (e.g. erythropoietin (EPO))
- Drugs that conceal pain (e.g. opiates)
- Drugs that are stimulant (e.g. amfetamines)
- Drugs that are relaxant (e.g. beta blockers)
- Drugs used to control weight (e.g. diuretics)
- Drugs that mask the presence of other drugs (e.g. diuretics).

Substances banned at all times include anabolic steroids and hormones including EPO, human growth hormone, insulin-like growth factor (IGF-1), human chorionic gonadotropin, and adrenocorticotropic hormone. In addition, some methods of performance enhancement are banned at all times and these include methods to enhance oxygen transfer such as blood doping and artificial oxygen carriers, chemical and physical manipulation (including tampering with samples and intravenous infusion), and gene doping.

Substances banned only in competition include stimulants such as amphetamines, ephedrine, and cocaine; opiates; cannabinoids; and glucocorticosteroids.

Other substances are banned only in particular sports. For example, alcohol is prohibited when competing in sports such as paragliding, skydiving, anything involving aircraft, archery, automobile sports, motorcycling, and power boating. A doping violation occurs at a blood alcohol concentration of 0.10 g/L or more. Beta blockers are prohibited in many sports where control of anxiety for motor coordination is required such as archery, automobile sports, motor cycling, billiards and snooker, darts, golf, shooting, ski jumping, freestyle skiing, and snowboarding.

Beta agonists such as salbutamol and formoterol have anabolic effects when administered in large doses. This is usually only possible by oral or intramuscular dosing and regular inhaled beta agonists to treat asthma or exercise-induced bronchospasm do not have this effect. Non-therapeutic use is defined as urine concentrations of 1000 ng/mL or more of salbutamol and 40 ng/mL or more of formoterol.

5.4 **Aetiology**

Biological, psychological, and social factors are all important in aetiology. Considering factors in these three areas is helpful in devising prevention strategies, informing social policy, and when formulating individual problems at the time of assessment.

5.4.1 **Biological**

Biological factors include genetics, gender (males are at higher risk), and a possible priming effect in maturing brains where drug exposure in adolescence increases later susceptibility to the effects of other drugs.

5.4.2 **Psychological**

Psychological stresses can lead to addiction problems and the 'stress/vulnerability model' of illness is useful in understanding how. At times of very high stress even the most resilient may have problems whilst at times of low stress it is only the most vulnerable who run into difficulty. Drug use is often immediately gratifying and therefore positively reinforced in preference to more adaptive but delayed ways of coping. Some personality traits increase risk, especially poor impulse control and risk-taking tendencies.

5.4.3 **Social**

Social factors are important too and substance misuse is associated with parental modelling, peer influences, poor family cohesion, deprivation, and poverty. Economic factors also come into play as the use of many drugs is sensitive to their cost and availability.

Aetiological factors in sportspeople mirror those in the wider population. Using the stress vulnerability model it is useful to consider an athlete's pre-existing vulnerability, and stresses that may trigger or maintain episodes. In each of these areas biological, social, or psychological factors may be important. Athletes can find themselves in a high-pressure environment where personality traits such as perfectionism, impulsivity, and novelty seeking may be more marked and increase vulnerability to substance misuse. Some may also work in a subculture where certain drugs (e.g. alcohol) are routinely used in team rituals and where a subculture of heavy use is endemic.

With regard to PEDs then, some aspects of the sports environment can promote use. Firstly and most obviously an athlete may make a conscious and considered decision to use illegal substances to enhance his or her performance in pursuit of success and wealth. Others may find themselves in an environment where use is prolific and accepted. They may find their sporting ideals subject to a process of attrition that leads them to consider doping simply to be competitive or to fit in. They may feel a strong sense of obligation to teammates and sponsors. These circumstances can lead to an ego-dystonic and reluctant although still conscious decision to dope. There will be some, perhaps used to obeying team orders or following the advice of coaches and others, who will take whatever supplements or substances are offered without question. Finally, there have also been undoubted instances where more malign coercion has been used in state-sponsored doping programmes.

Surveys of elite athletes report the following reasons for using PEDs:

- Achievement of athletic success by improved performance
- Financial gain
- Improving recovery
- Prevention of nutritional deficiencies
- Others use them.

5.5 **Prevalence and patterns of use**

5.5.1 **General population**

Almost 25% of the adult population in the European Union (over 80 million adults) is estimated to have used illicit drugs at some point in their lives, in most cases cannabis. Levels of lifetime use vary considerably between countries from around one-third of adults in the United Kingdom, Denmark, and France to less than one in ten in Bulgaria, Greece, and Hungary (The European Monitoring Centre for Drugs and Drug Addiction, 2014). In the United States, the Annual National Survey on Drug Use and Health (NSDUH) from 2013, estimate that 9.4% (24.6 million) had used an illicit drug in the month prior to the survey with cannabis the most commonly used drug.

It is estimated that 25% of 15–16-year-olds have used an illicit drug and cannabis is again the most likely drug to be used by all age groups.

Cocaine is the most commonly used illicit stimulant in Europe but the prevalence is declining. The illicit use of opiates remains responsible for a disproportionately large share of the morbidity and mortality and the main opiate remains heroin. However, opioids other than heroin (including buprenorphine and fentanyl) are of increasing concern.

In recent years, there has been a startling rise in the use of novel psychoactive substances (NPSs—also known as legal highs). These are synthetic substances that mimic or claim to mimic the effects of drugs. They are ever evolving (81 new psychoactive substances were notified to the European Union in 2013 compared to 24 in 2009). They are synthesized to evade detection and legal prohibition and most are not controlled under the Misuse of Drugs Act although some have been banned (e.g. mephedrone in the United Kingdom).

NPSs include synthetic cannabinoids (often natural herbs sprayed with chemicals) also known as Spice drugs and a group of drugs known as cathinones which mimic the effects of stimulants like cocaine. Concentration (strength) is variable and effects cannot be predicted. They are usually marked as 'not for human consumption' and labelled as items such bath salts, research chemicals, or plant food. They may produce more potent effects than their natural counterparts with greater psychological and physical harm and can induce feelings of anxiety, panic, paranoia, and can cause psychosis.

5.5.2 **Sports**

The pattern of substance misuse varies in several respects when misuse within sport is compared to misuse in the general population. Most obviously the use of drugs for performance enhancement is commoner in this group. However, it is a misconception that PED use is limited to the elite athlete population. This has distracted attention from PED as a public health issue and there are an estimated 3 million PED users in the United States alone (more than have type 1 diabetes or HIV infection). Widespread use of PEDs is a relatively recent phenomenon and as a consequence the majority of users are under the age of 50. This means that the full scope of long-term effects of PEDs is yet to be determined.

Alcohol, caffeine, nicotine, and to a lesser extent cannabis are the most common substances of misuse in community samples and this largely holds true within sports too. However, serious problems of dependence are relatively less common and binge use (especially of alcohol) may be more common at certain times such as in the off-season, as part of team rituals, and to celebrate victory or deal with defeat.

A pattern of association can emerge where some drugs are more likely to be used alongside others. For example, misuse of alcohol, nicotine, and cannabis may co-occur and anabolic steroids are frequently used with other drugs that promote muscle growth. Some athletes who use stimulants during training and competition to increase energy and improve concentration may fall into a pattern of using hypnotics or alcohol to relax afterwards.

In contact and collision sports where injuries are regular and frequent, pain management can be problematic with players eager to return to play at the earliest opportunity. In this scenario opiate use (prescribed or illicit) can escalate and opiate dependence is an important and often unrecognized consequence. In sports where stimulants are used there is a risk of athletes progressing from the legal use of energy drinks and caffeine to more illicit substances. In these sports it is also possible that athletes may seek prescriptions for stimulants normally used to treat attention deficit hyperactivity disorder (ADHD) (see Chapter 6). A diagnosis of ADHD is made largely on self-reported symptoms or those observed by others. It is recommended that the diagnosis is not made without careful consideration, and that the TUE assessor is competent and proficient to make the diagnosis.

In 2010, WADA screened over quarter of a million specimens at 35 accredited laboratories worldwide. There were 4820 (1.9%) 'adverse atypical findings'. The most commonly detected substances within the adverse findings were anabolic agents (60.8%), stimulants (10.2%), cannabinoids (9.6%), and diuretic and other masking agents (7.1%).

The true prevalence of doping in elite sports is unknown as quite naturally athletes are reluctant to disclose their use when surveyed and testing procedures will only uncover a minority of cases. Questionnaires that use the randomized response technique estimate that 14–39% of adult elite athletes are intentionally doping. This technique is an established method for asking embarrassing or threatening questions while allowing the respondents to answer honestly. The technique determines the rate of 'honest dopers' who admit their use and extrapolates this using data on positive test rates to estimate the actual prevalence of all athletes who are doping.

A survey of adolescent athletes revealed 1.2% who reported using doping agents at least once in the preceding 6 months. This rate rose to 3.0% when the same group were resurveyed 4 years later. Of those who had used, 4% reported a related health problem but 44% had won at least one sporting event attributed to the drug. Whilst athletes acknowledge that doping is cheating, unhealthy, and risky its effectiveness is also widely recognized.

5.6 Exercise addiction

Whilst 'addiction' is commonly used when describing those who exercise excessively or compulsively it is not an entirely appropriate term for several reasons. Those who exercise to excess may experience restlessness and anxiety associated with craving if denied the opportunity to exercise but this is invariably mild compared to the experience of alcohol or opiate dependence. Tolerance, too, is unlikely to develop. Nonetheless there are some who undoubtedly spend a great deal of time exercising or recovering from exercise at the expense of other roles and activities. They may also experience some physical harm from the intensity of their activity and especially from the desire to continue even when injured.

Likewise, 'excessive' may not be an entirely fitting description. It implies that exercise is judged by its quantity. Sportspeople spend large amounts of time exercising, preparing to exercise, or in recovery. In most cases this will be entirely functional, motivated by a desire to improve and regulated by a training programme. Other motivations may lie behind exercising behaviour. When these are considered then compulsive exercise appears the most apt description to capture the nature of the desire to continue when it would be logical to rest (e.g. when injured) and the anxiety experienced if activities are curtailed.

There is likely to be a biological component to compulsive exercise that results from the release of endogenous opioids after exercise and that enhance mood. Many will also feel compelled to exercise as a way of avoiding a negative mood and may lack other, more helpful, means of regulating unpleasant emotional states. There may be a rigid style of thinking where inflexible rules govern behaviour. Exercise may also be a means of weight control in those who experience persistent dissatisfaction with their perception of their physical appearance.

Assessment of compulsive exercise involves a careful enquiry about these factors. If compulsive exercise appears secondary to, for example, a depressive illness or an eating disorder then the treatment is as for the underlying condition. Otherwise determining the athlete's stage of change and readiness to change behaviour is important and motivational techniques can be employed if necessary. If the athlete lacks other emotional regulation techniques then interventions should focus on developing these using, for example, cognitive behavioural therapy or another of the techniques described in Chapters 1 and 2.

5.7 Screening and early detection

5.7.1 Drugs and alcohol

With respect to the usual common substances of misuse there is no substitute for an aware and vigilant clinician when trying to spot a problem at an early stage. Team doctors should be alert to the possibility of misuse of common substances but especially alcohol, stimulants, misused and illicit analgesics (especially opiates), and hypnotics including benzodiazepines. They should be aware of the common warning signs of a problem such as a drop in performance, mood changes, interpersonal problems, and social withdrawal. Other members of the support team can also be taught to look for early signs as they are often in a position to detect difficulties at an earlier stage.

Screening tools for assessment, severity, and monitoring of symptoms all help to inform treatment and are increasingly used.

CAGE is the basic and opportunistic screening tool for alcohol, this asks about whether an individual has tried to Cut down their use, felt Annoyed by people criticizing their drinking, experienced Guilt about their drinking or ever needed an Eye-opener. However, the gold standard is the AUDIT (the Alcohol Use Disorders Identification Test) which is validated across cultures and also gives an indication of severity with ten questions and a maximum score of 40. This can help inform management. Scores of 8–15 indicate hazardous drinking (consumption which increases the risk of harm) and should be managed with simple structured advice. Scores of 16–19 indicate harmful drinking (ICD–10) and indicate the need for brief interventions and follow up, and score of over 20 suggest possible dependence which should be diagnosed with referral on to specialist services.

Similar screening tools exist for drugs, for example, the National Institute for Drug Abuse Drug Use Screening Tool is available at http://www.drugabuse.gov. It evaluates current and lifetime use and ascribes a risk score of low, moderate, or high to determine the need for interventions.

The Severity of Alcohol Dependence Questionnaire gives an indication of the severity of dependence and will again inform management, for example, of the need for alcohol detoxification.

The Clinical Institute Withdrawal of Alcohol Scale revised (CIWA-Ar) gives an indication of the severity of alcohol withdrawal and will inform the management of the detoxification.

The Alcohol Problems Questionnaire is used to assess both the nature and extent of problems arising from alcohol.

5.7.2 Performance-enhancing drugs

Often the first sign that a PED is being used is when an athlete tests positive in competition or during a random out-of-competition test. Sport takes an approach of 'strict liability' (the athlete alone is responsible for what is found in his/her blood or urine) and the likely response is a punitive one that may remove the athlete from his or her support network. This can be a significant obstacle to providing any necessary psychiatric expertise and support to a problem user.

Each potential PED demands that a new test is developed and validated. The athlete passport is promoted as a potential alternative to blood and urine testing for doping products. The athlete passport records and reports a series of physiological parameters over the athlete's career and provides evidence of the stability of that individual's physiology. Multiple measures are recorded serially. Inconsistencies and fluctuations will alert to the possibility of a PED being used. The blood module of the passport aims to detect blood doping, whilst the steroid module will provide evidence of anabolic steroid use, and the endocrine module will identify anomalies of growth hormones or other growth factors (e.g. IGF-1).

The common side effects and adverse effects of PEDs are summarized in Table 5.1.

Table 5.1 Common side effects and adverse effects of PEDs

Performance-enhancing drug	Side effects
Anabolic agents	Cardiomyopathy, atherosclerosis, hepatic dysfunction, aplastic anaemia hypercoagulopathy, psychiatric disturbance including psychosis, depression, and aggression
Peptide hormones, mimetics, and analogues	Acne, abnormal growth, cerebrovascular accident, hypertension, diabetes, and arthritis
Blood doping—use of infusion (often autologous) to increase red cell mass and hence oxygen carrying capacity. EPO.	Allergic reactions, risk of blood borne viruses, e.g. HIV Hypertension, overload of circulatory system, and renal failure
Artificial oxygen carriers and plasma expanders	As for blood doping and iron overload
Opiates including opiate analgesics	Mood disturbances, vomiting, constipation, respiratory depression and arrest, hypotension, addiction
Stimulants	Increased heart rate, anxiety, hypertension
Beta blockers	Gastric irritation, depression, fatigue, sexual dysfunction, bronchospasm
Diuretics	Hypotension, dehydration, headaches, nausea, muscle cramps

Reproduced from *Vignettes of Research*, 1(4), Kumar S, Performance Enhancing Drugs in Sport. p. 164–169, Copyright (2013), with permission from *Vignettes of Research*.

5.8 **Assessment**

A persistent but non-judgemental approach is required for successful exploration of problems that the athlete may be very reluctant to disclose. This is in part related to readiness to change and fear of the consequences of disclosure. The biopsychosocial model of understanding problems that prevails in psychiatric practice is especially helpful for exploring and understanding complex problems of substance misuse and in most cases is to be preferred to a moral model which frames addiction as a result of human weakness.

The biopsychosocial model allows exploration of the contribution of factors in these three domains. Factors such as genetic predisposition, the neurobiology of reward systems, drug dependence, and withdrawal; the contribution of an individual's psychology (personality traits, low mood); and the social context in which abuse can be triggered, nurtured, and sustained are all addressed by this model. A detailed formulation will also consider pre-existing vulnerability, trigger events, and maintaining factors in each of these three domains.

The assessment will include several areas of enquiry:

1. History:
   - A detailed chronology of pattern of substance use, previous symptoms, diagnosis, and treatment
   - Include the period before the onset of substance abuse as well as periods of extended abstinence
   - Antecedents and context
   - Triggers—onset and development of misuse
   - Maintaining factors including a social context that may allow the problem to go undetected or even to flourish
   - Symptoms of tolerance and withdrawal.

2. Problems:
   - Secondary problems such as relationship, financial, and performance difficulties
   - Screen for any co-morbid problems (e.g. depression).

3. Readiness:
   - Try and understand the function of the drug/substance of abuse for that individual
   - Determine stage of change for each problem
   - A description of current strengths and limitations that may enhance or inhibit an individual's ability to follow the recommended treatment regimen
   - Identify external contingencies that might help to promote treatment adherence (e.g. family support systems or incentives such as voucher schemes to encourage treatment adherence).

4. Immediate needs:
   - What are the immediate needs?
   - What are the individual's priorities?
   - What support networks are available (especially important for younger substance misusers)?

5. Contract:
   - At engagement, determine what the client is aiming to achieve
   - What specific services are necessary to achieve these aims?
     - Psychological input/therapy
     - Pharmacological management
     - Other supports
   - How will outcomes be measured?
   - What follow-up is need and how will progress be monitored?
   - Agree a treatment contract.

The stages of change model described by Prochaska and DiClemente (see Figure 4.2 in Chapter 4) represents a series of psychological shifts that are experienced when modifying chronic behavioural patterns. These are important to understand as they have implications for the likelihood of successful change which depends on the individual's stage within the model. The model is cyclical and allows for relapses into former behaviours and movement forwards and backwards through the stages. Assessing the stage of change can inform the natures of interventions that follow. For example, a focus on motivational work for those who are contemplating, on goal setting for those in preparatory stages, and on detoxification for those in determination and action stages.

5.9 **Treatment**

A stepped approach to treatment, reflecting both the nature and severity of the substance misuse as well as the needs and wishes of the patient, is essential. Reflecting the biopsychosocial model, treatment usually comprises psychosocial interventions with or without pharmacotherapy. For those patients who meet the criteria for harmful use (ICD-10) but do not meet the criteria for a dependence syndrome, psychosocial approaches are the mainstay of treatment and pharmacological treatments less applicable.

Harm minimization is an ethos that runs throughout treatment, rather than treatment per se. It is a principle that acknowledges that not everybody is ready to stop using substances and aims to minimize the harm arising from use, for example, through the provision of sterile equipment for injecting.

Further aims of treatment include the maintenance of abstinence (e.g. relapse prevention) and the prevention and treatment of complications (e.g. thiamine for prevention of Wernicke's encephalopathy and vaccination for hepatitis A and B).

Screening and assessment are the first opportunities to provide treatment that may take the form of a brief intervention. Brief interventions can be offered in any setting and are opportunistic, varying in length from 10–45 minutes. They focus on motivation to change behaviour, explore ambivalence about substance use and treatment, and provide non-judgemental feedback.

In all cases, families and carers should be encouraged to be involved in care and treatment and be offered self-help and contact with support groups.

In addition, all people who misuse substances should be given information on the value and availability of support networks and self-help groups, for example, Alcoholics Anonymous and Narcotics Anonymous (these are abstinence based and work to the principles of the 12-step programme). SMART recovery is a four-point programme (building and maintaining motivation; coping with urges; managing thoughts, feelings, and behaviours; and living a balanced life) with face-to-face meetings, daily online meetings, and chat rooms.

Contingency management, based on the principles of operant conditioning, is a process that attempts to modify behaviour through the use of positive reinforcements when the desired behaviour is achieved, for example, vouchers for negative drug tests. There is evidence for the use of contingency management in the reduction of illicit drug use and the promotion of engagement with services, particularly for people receiving methadone maintenance and primary stimulant users. It is also used within other public health settings such as smoking cessation and weight loss clinics; however, its use remains controversial with the general public.

5.9.1 **Alcohol**

Interventions for harmful drinking and mild alcohol dependence (scoring 8–19 on AUDIT) should include a psychological therapy, for example, cognitive behavioural therapy, behavioural couples therapy (to patients with a partner willing to participate in treatment), or social network and environment-based therapies focused on alcohol-related cognitions, behaviour, problems, and social networks.

Nalmefene (a competitive antagonist at the opioid receptor) is recommended as a possible treatment for people with mild alcohol dependence and no physical withdrawal symptoms who do not need to stop drinking straight away or stop drinking completely. Again it needs to be delivered in conjunction with psychosocial interventions and there is no evidence that it is superior to placebo without these.

Patients who are judged to be alcohol dependent (scoring more than 20 on the AUDIT) may need a medically assisted withdrawal. The setting for this will depend on the severity of dependence, physical and mental co-morbidity, and social support. Longer-acting benzodiazepines, for example, chlordiazepoxide or diazepam, are used as the preferred medication.

For community-assisted alcohol detoxification, fixed-dose regimens are used. Those receiving 24-hour care, for example, hospital in-patients, can be given a symptom-triggered regimen where severity of withdrawal (measured with a rating scale, e.g. the CIWA-Ar) determines the dose of medication. Thiamine (oral or parenteral depending on severity of dependence and co-morbidity) should be offered to all undergoing alcohol detoxification to prevent Wernicke's encephalopathy and Korsakoff's syndrome.

After medically assisted alcohol withdrawal, those with moderate and severe alcohol dependence should be offered the anticraving agents acamprosate or naltrexone (as an adjunct to psychosocial interventions). Acamprosate inhibits glutaminergic NMDA receptor function *in vitro* although the mechanism of action *in vivo* is not entirely clear. It may also have a neuroprotective effect during detoxification. Naltrexone is an opiate antagonist purported to reduce the pleasurable effects of alcohol by blocking the effects of opioids released by alcohol that enhance dopamine release in the mesolimbic system. Both have been shown to be more effective than placebo across a range of drinking outcome measures but usually in conjunction with psychosocial interventions.

Disulfiram has been used for many years to promote abstinence and again can be used post detoxification in combination with a psychological intervention. It induces an unpleasant reaction if taken with alcohol (flushing, nausea, headache, palpitations) by blocking the metabolism of alcohol, resulting in a build-up in acetaldehyde. Witnessing the consumption of disulfiram is important and when prescribed without supervision, disulfiram is no better than basic support.

5.9.2 **Tobacco**

In many countries, tobacco use has declined in popularity and acceptability in recent years. Its effects on the cardiovascular and respiratory systems are such that use by athletes is lower than in the general population although chewing tobacco is popular in some sports (notably baseball). Nicotine is a highly addictive drug and interventions to reduce and stop tobacco use are widely available. Self-help materials can be augmented by behavioural support including goal setting and self-monitoring. This can be supplemented by nicotine-containing products used as tobacco replacements. These come in many forms including inhalators, transdermal patches, nasal and oral sprays, gum, and sublingual tablets. Prescribed medications are also available. Varenicline is a partial agonist at nicotine receptors and reduces withdrawal symptoms whilst making smoking less rewarding. Bupropion is also effective in reducing nicotine cravings and withdrawal symptoms.

5.9.3 **Opiate dependence**

Methadone, buprenorphine, and Suboxone® (buprenorphine and naloxone in a 4:1 combination) are used for both opiate detoxification and maintenance therapy. They are long acting which allows for once-daily dosing and hence supervised consumption within the community pharmacy setting. All reduce opiate withdrawals and craving. All should be used within a programme of structured psychosocial interventions. Following detoxification, naltrexone may be used to both block the effects of any relapse into opiate use and also reduce craving.

5.9.4 **Stimulants**

Both cocaine and amphetamine have powerful effects on brain dopamine. They produce a state of elation, euphoria, and excitement accompanied by alertness. The mainstay of management is with psychological approaches. Sedatives such as benzodiazepines can be employed to reduce anxiety and agitation in the acute phase of detoxification but caution is needed as they are also associated with dependency and often misused. Antidepressants can be considered if there is co-morbid depression.

5.9.5 **Anabolic steroids**

It is unclear whether or not anabolic steroids produce a physical dependence. ICD-10 categorizes them as 'non-dependence producing substances' whilst DSM-5 raises the possibility that there is potential for dependence. They can certainly create psychological dependence and are associated with psychiatric morbidity including depression and anxiety that may require treatment.

5.9.6 **Residential rehabilitation**

For people who are unable to attain stability within the community setting despite optimized treatment, then residential rehabilitation may be considered. The focus is on health, personal, and social functioning and enhanced quality of life. There are a number of different therapeutic approaches but most are abstinence based and run to a 12-step programme or therapeutic approach. The evidence for therapeutic communities, however, remains inconclusive.

5.10 **Summary/conclusion**

Psychiatric expertise is helpful in understanding the complexities of substance misuse within sport. This is not restricted to the usual problems of substance misuse and dependence seen elsewhere in society, although this is clearly important. Athletes need good treatment and support and don't always get this. The knowledge and skills of a psychiatrist also extend to understanding how and why athletes come to use PEDs. With this understanding, appropriate support and treatment can be offered. Rehabilitation, recovery, and the prospect of a life beyond drug use can be added to the existing portfolio of responses for an athlete who dopes. Testing, no matter how frequent or reliable, targets doping behaviours rather than athlete attitudes.

There are arguments that the legalization of drugs in sport would make it fairer and safer. The welfare (not the performance) of the athlete is the primary concern of any medical professional. If a drug does not expose an athlete to excessive risk might it be safer to allow its use but aim to reduce the harm by offering medical support? This has parallels with 'harm reduction' methods used in some addictions and indeed needles are available via needle exchanges to recreational anabolic steroid users. However, most healthcare professionals who work in sport are aware not just of the controversies in condoning the use of substances with no health benefit and likely harm but also of the benefits of sports participation for individuals, within societies and across cultures. Many would therefore view support for the use of PEDs with no medical indication as a violation of sporting ethics. Current regulations and guidance is also very clear. In the United Kingdom, doctors who deviate from General Medical Council guidance and prescribe with the intention of improving sporting performance risk losing their registration.

Case study 1

A 23-year-old footballer consulted the club doctor accompanied by his wife. He had recently been fined for missing preseason training sessions and had been excluded from a preseason tour as a result. His wife reported that problem drinking was the primary reason for his behaviour. She had been prompting him to seek help repeatedly over a 2–3-month period but he had always refused until his recent fine and exclusion.

He described drinking beer at a local club in the later afternoon until early evening and then several glasses of vodka in the late evening at home (sometime 20–25 units per day in total). He had been drinking at this level for about a year. He was sleeping poorly and had recently begun to have 2 glasses of vodka in the morning to 'straighten himself out' if he were shaky and retching. He had little appetite and had lost weight. There were frequent arguments with his wife.

At assessment he described how he had been brought up in a teetotal family in rural Ireland but had started drinking with older players when he left home and joined the club's youth academy at the age of 16. He signed a lucrative contract at the age of 18 and had a large disposal income as well as copious free time that he spent in a local snooker hall drinking with his teammates.

He agreed that he now wanted to address his problems and work to re-establish his place in the team. He was prescribed a fixed-dose chlordiazepoxide reduction regimen over 5 days and oral thiamine tablets. He and his wife were offered and attended for 12 sessions of behavioural couples therapy. He joined a local support group (Alcoholics Anonymous). There he met a former player, now retired, who had been abstinent for 8 years and who encouraged him to spend his afternoons helping with a local youth sports project. He was prescribed daily acamprosate and remains abstinent 18 months later.

Case study 2

A team doctor was asked by his physiotherapy colleague to see a 28-year-old discus thrower and a psychiatric assessment was then requested to evaluate the use of opiate analgesics by the thrower.

The athlete had sustained a shoulder injury when weight-lifting a few weeks before his competitive season started. He rested for a week and took some OTC non-steroidal anti-inflammatories. His pain settled but he sustained a re-injury in his first competition. He saw a physiotherapist but was poorly adherent to the rehabilitation programme by overusing his throwing arm and lifting more than recommended in the gym. He continued with anti-inflammatories, which had now been prescribed, and in addition began using opiate analgesics (codeine phosphate) in steadily increasing does of up to 120 mg daily that he obtained from a private general practitioner. Later he began using illicitly obtained tramadol (up to 200 mg daily) in addition. The physiotherapist had become concerned when he requested a steroid injection and further enquiry revealed the opiate misuse.

After the psychiatric assessment a joint appointment was arranged with athlete, coach, physiotherapist, team doctor, and psychiatrist. A clear description of the injury, its severity and likely recovery course was discussed. This allowed all to agree to a rehabilitation plan that would give hope for a return in time for some important end-of-season events. Buprenorphine was suggested to help with cravings and withdrawal symptoms during an opiate detoxification programme. The athlete was wary of this approach and instead a stabilization and reduction plan was implemented. Opiate use was stabilized over a 4-week period using codeine only (at a dose of 240 mg daily) and then a reduction regimen proceeded over a further 4-week period.

Further reading

American Psychiatric Association (2013). *Diagnostic and Statistical Manual of Mental Disorders* (5th ed.). Washington, DC: American Psychiatric Association.

Babor, T.F., Higgins-Biddle, J.C., Saunders, J.B., and Grant, M.G. (2001). *AUDIT: The Alcohol Use Disorders Identification Test: Guidelines for Use in Primary Health* Care (2nd ed.). *Geneva*: World Health Organization.

Ghodse, A.H. (2010). *Ghodse's Drugs and Addictive Behaviour: A Guide to Treatment* (4th ed.). Cambridge: Cambridge University Press.

Jarvis, T., Tebbutt, J., and Mattick, R.P. (2005). *Treatment Approaches for Alcohol and Drug Dependence: An Introductory Guide*. Chichester: John Wiley & Sons.

Kumar, S. (2013). Performance enhancing drugs in sport. *Vignettes Res* 1(4):164–9.

Lingford-Hughes, A.R., Welch, S., Peters, L., and Nutt, D.J. (2012). BAP updated guidelines: evidence-based guidelines for the pharmacological management of substance abuse, harmful use, addiction and comorbidity: recommendations from BAP. *J Psychopharmacol* 26(7):899–952.

Mayfield, D., McLeod, G., and Hall, P. (1974). The CAGE Questionnaire: validation of a new alcoholism screening instrument. *Am J Psychiatry* 131(10):1121–3.

McDuff, D.R. and Baron, D. (2005). Substance use in athletics: a sports psychiatry perspective. *Clin Sports Med* 24:885–97.

Morente-Sanchez, J. and Zabala, M. (2013). Doping in sport: a review of elite athletes' attitudes, beliefs and knowledge. *Sports Med* 43:395–411.

Morse, E.D. (2013). Substance use in athletes. In Baron, D.A., Reardon, C.L., and Baron, S.H. (Eds.), *Clinical Sports Psychiatry: An International Perspective* (pp. 1–12). Oxford: Wiley.

Peterson, T. and McBride, A. (2002). *Working with Substance Misusers: A Guide to Theory and Practice*. London: Routledge.

Prochaska, J. and Diclemente, C. (1983). Stages and processes of self-change in smoking: toward an integrative model of change. *J Consult Clin Psychol* 5:390–5.

Selzer, M.L. (1971). The Michigan alcoholism screening test: the quest for a new diagnostic instrument. *Am J Psychiatry* 127(12):1653–8.

Skinner, H.A. (1982). The Drug Abuse Screening test. *Addictive Behav* 7(4):363–71.

Strachan, A. (2012). Substance misuse in sport: current controversies and surrounding issues. *Biomed Scientist* June:334–9.

Sullivan, J.T., Sykara, K., Schneiderman, J., Naranjo, C.A., and Sellers, E.M. (1989). Assessment of alcohol withdrawal: the revised Clinical Institute Withdrawal Assessment for Alcohol Scale (CIWA-Ar). *Br J Addict* 84:1353–7.

Wesson, D.R. and Ling, W. (2003). The Clinical Opiate Withdrawal Scale (COWS). *J Psychoactive Drugs* 35(2):253–9.

World Health Organization (1999). *International Statistical Classification of Diseases and Related Health Problems 10th Revision.* Geneva: World Health Organization.

Website

World Anti-Doping Agency: https://www.wada-ama.org

Chapter 6

Attention deficit hyperactivity disorder

Paul McArdle

Key points

- Attention deficit hyperactivity disorder (ADHD) is a relatively common condition that emerges early in development and may last into adulthood.
- Sufferers struggle to concentrate, especially on abstract tasks that require mental effort, to sit still, and to foresee negative consequences of actions.
- It is crucial for coaches and others to spot ADHD, often aided by online and other screening questionnaires.
- Once the diagnosis is confirmed by an expert, behavioural techniques may be transformative. These should emphasize routine, structure, and, crucially, simplicity and clarity of instructions, with checks to ensure they are comprehensible to the subject.

6.1 Introduction

Attention deficit hyperactivity disorder (ADHD) is characterized by hyperactivity, inattention, and impulsivity. In addition, it is necessary that these features are judged to be:

1. Out of keeping with the person's age
2. Evident in a number of settings
3. Impairing social, educational, or occupational activities
4. Present before the age of 12 years.

The clinical features fall into two broad groups. There are signs of marked inattention/distractibility accompanied by hyperactivity with impulsivity.

Inattention and distractibility are often most apparent in settings requiring active attention such as at school, with homework, or in the work place. In these settings, an inability to engage in effortful tasks is conspicuous. Some tasks such as playing on computer games with rapid feedback on performance may be unimpaired and do not rule out the diagnosis.

Inability to concentrate can make it difficult to follow complex sequences. This may be evident on the sports field and one football-playing sufferer described how 'the ball will be passed to me and I might be lookin' in the trees or somethin' and then just everybody jumps down my throat'. In solitary sports and pursuits, where planning may be crucial, there is also a disadvantage to sufferers.

The second set of symptoms is in the realm of 'hyperactivity/impulsivity'. These features often wane with maturation into adulthood. They may be most noticeable in situations that require calm. Impulsivity may be noticed in an inability to see consequences. An ability to instinctively evaluate what will happen next may be lacking in the child caught in a school fracas from which others, perhaps more guilty, fled in time or in the player who fouls right in front of the referee.

6.2 **Diagnosis**

The diagnosis is usually made by interviewing the patient and someone familiar with their development, often a family member. Questions focus on current symptoms in the two realms of inattention/distractibility and hyperactivity/impulsivity. It is important to consider how they have evolved during the patient's early life as it is a necessary criterion that symptoms were first present before the age of 12 years.

A formal diagnosis is usually made based on clinical findings, reports, and observations by an experienced clinician able to distinguish ADHD from other disorders that have overlapping features. These include autism, learning disability, and perhaps bipolar disorder. There are no tests that confirm or refute the diagnosis and observations in a clinical interview or in psychological testing where the individual is often on best behaviour, can be misleading.

In sport, establishing the diagnosis is important as treatments may include otherwise banned stimulants. A special Therapeutic Use Exemption (TUE) can be granted if it can be firmly established that ADHD is present (Box 6.1). This requires that the diagnosis is made by a specialist (some sports say two independent specialists if the diagnosis is made for the first time in an adult) and that there is evidence of standardized criteria being applied, for example, from the International Classification of Diseases, version 10 (ICD-10) or Diagnostic and Statistical Manual of Mental Disorders, fifth edition (DSM-5).

Structured interviews are available but can be time-consuming although they do ensure a standardized approach. As they are based on established diagnostic criteria they may add little to the assessment of an expert. The Child and Adolescent Psychiatric Assessment (CAPA) is semi-structured, covers all diagnoses, and can be administered by a clinician trained in its use. It is based on self-reports augmented by information from parents. There is no requirement to include information from school teachers (which can often be very valuable in establishing a diagnosis). The Diagnostic Interview for ADHD in Adults (DIVA—http://www.psyq.nl/files/1263005/DIVA_2_EN.pdf) is based on DSM criteria and uses self-report and where possible information from a partner or other family member. It takes around 90 minutes to complete.

6.2.1 **Other features**

ADHD is also associated with deficits in language development, often related to short working memory as long sentences are not held in mind long enough to be deciphered. Children learn to pretend they have understood when they have not. Non-compliant behaviour may resemble defiance but is actually incomprehension.

Faced with constant reprimands for distracted behaviour, frequent underperformance in school, and incomprehension of the spoken and written word in a highly

---

Box 6.1 Features and symptoms of ADHD

Main features
- Early onset (symptoms present before age 12)
- Pervasive over many situations
- Persistent over time:
  - Through school years and even into adult life (although many affected individuals show a gradual improvement in activity and attention with maturation)
- Overactive, poorly modulated behaviour:
  - Reckless and impulsive, prone to accidents, and find themselves in disciplinary trouble because of unthinking (rather than deliberately defiant) breaches of rules
  - Relationships with adults are often socially disinhibited with a lack of normal caution and reserve
- Marked inattention and lack of persistent task involvement
- Unpopular with other children and may become isolated
- Cognitive impairment is common:
  - Specific delays in motor and language development are disproportionately frequent

Other symptoms
- Wastes or mismanages time
- Cannot work unless under a deadline
- Cannot complete tasks on time
- Lacks self-discipline
- Bores easily
- Others keep life in order

- Trouble planning ahead
- Difficulty prioritizing work
- Trouble keeping track of multiple things
- Remembers details, not main idea
- Easily overwhelmed
- Mood changes frequently.

---

verbal culture, their disappointment in themselves can be intense. Not surprisingly the prevalence of depression and anxiety among adults with ADHD is twice that in the general population.

ADHD is often associated with difficulties in maintaining friendships, difficulty seeing others' perspective, and comments that seem insensitive. Other autistic-like difficulties such as distress at unexpected change are present. In sport, this may appear when asked to play out of position or after being substituted early.

6.2.2 **Aetiology**

ADHD may represent persistence into adolescence and adulthood of behaviour usually seen in younger children. Brain scans show that the normal maturation of grey matter, with the pruning of redundant brain cells during adolescence, is delayed in ADHD.

The frontal cortex and contiguous structures (linked to ADHD) can mature with time and perhaps half of children with ADHD will grow out of it. The other half have symptoms that persist into adulthood and some may never quite catch up.

The theory that the core of ADHD is a deficit in executive function is clinically meaningful and has explanatory power. Executive functions are responsible for goal directed behaviour and for self-regulation organized by the person's aims and purposefulness. The frontal cortex and related brain areas are the anatomical counterparts of these functions.

The mind management model ('chimp paradox') described in Chapter 2 is a simple and accessible way of understanding this. It may be helpful for those who work in sport and are already familiar with the 'chimp' model. The executive functions located in the frontal lobes and related areas equate to 'the human'. The 'chimp' is located in the limbic system and related structures and is responsible for emotional and instinctive responses. In ADHD, 'the chimp' is more likely to be active because of deficits in self-control associated with frontal impairments. Affected individuals in effect lack a behavioural endoskeleton to structure their lives. This may well be the key immaturity that resolves in some but persists into adulthood in others.

There is substantial evidence that ADHD is largely genetically determined. This view has come to supersede the minimal brain damage concept, that children through a difficult birth might have lasting subtle defects. Nevertheless, premature babies and those with early severe psychosocial deprivation can display ADHD-like disruptive behaviours. Some also cite the influence of environmental toxins such as lead or alcohol, especially during pregnancy.

These are not the only hypothesized ways of understanding ADHD. It has also been described as an unusual pattern of subjective reward where small and immediate rewards are strongly preferred over larger but delayed rewards (aversion to delay) or that the clinical features of ADHD simply represent the statistical extremes of normal temperament.

Developmental delay or brain injury hypotheses view ADHD as fundamentally a vulnerability. Indeed, children with ADHD perform poorly at school, have friendship problems, are at risk of substance misuse, crime, educational failure, road traffic accidents, and premature mortality. Because of the disadvantages in our culture associated with ADHD, sufferers encounter serial defeats throughout development. They learn from school that there is no point in trying as failure is inevitable. This can resemble passive defiance.

6.2.3 **Can ADHD be an advantage?**

Formal compulsory schooling for all, where children have to sit in classrooms, focusing on abstractions such as reading and numbers, often with minimal immediate feedback, is a cultural innovation of the past 150 years. For those with ADHD, this experience may be particularly disadvantageous and exacerbated by the loss of freedom to play and explore experienced by children since the 1970s.

ADHD elicits hostility in our culture that contributes to further disruptive behaviour. This may not be the case everywhere and may not have occurred in the distant past. It has been argued that sensation seeking and courage consequent on the impulsive person's failure to consider negative consequences would have aided survival in groups of migrating hunters. In hunter-gatherer societies, ADHD could have been an asset.

6.2.4 **Genetics**

The *DRD4* gene codes for D4 dopamine receptors in the brain (dopamine is a neuro-transmitter that is important in ADHD). It has several different alleles and the 7R allele is associated with ADHD. This same allele is reported to offer an advantage among certain nomadic men in northern Kenya but a disadvantage for their settled counter-parts. It is hypothesized that the shorter attention spans associated with the 7R allele support learning in a dynamic environment (without schools) where the same attribute interferes with classroom learning in settled communities. It is further speculated that 7R+ boys might be more effective in defending against livestock raiders and develop a reputation as fearless warriors but are less suited to a settled agricultural life.

6.2.5 **Sport**

Among American footballers in the National Football League (NFL) the prevalence of previously diagnosed ADHD is 7%. This is approximately double the rate in the general adult population and suggests that ADHD is not a disadvantage in this set-ting. An association between attention deficit/learning disability and poorer verbal and visual memory has been found but no association with speed and reaction time in this population.

There is also a link between ADHD and sensation seeking, a personality trait com-mon among people who engage in contact and extreme sports. Such a person only feels fully engaged when immersed in exciting, potentially dangerous activity. In our culture, these traits may also translate into crime, substance misuse, road traffic colli-sions, and other accidents.

6.3 **Screening**

It appears likely that coaches and other professionals who work in sport will meet young players with ADHD and so they need to know how to spot a potential problem and then know how to get the best from these players. Whilst many adults will have grown out of historical ADHD this is by no means universal. In addition, there is good evidence that ADHD is underdiagnosed and this is important for two reasons. Firstly, a coach may be an excellent witness to features of ADHD and able to assist an expert in making the diagnosis. Secondly, a coach may find him/herself unknowingly managing an individual with the condition.

A useful guide is to consider possible ADHD if the individual:

• has ever been excluded from school

• seems of average ability but did badly in exams

• seems a bit anti-authority

• is typically distracted or even disruptive in teaching sessions.

Screening tools for ADHD in adults are available and can be offered by members of the athlete's medical support team to prompt and inform expert evaluation.

The Adult ADHD Self-Report Scale (ASRS) is an 18-item, self-report questionnaire based on DSM criteria. It is essentially a symptom checklist that also rates symptom frequency (http://www.hcp.med.harvard.edu/ncs/ftpdir/adhd/18Q_ASRS_English.pdf).

The diagnosis can only be confirmed by an experienced expert using standard and accepted criteria. This involves a detailed clinical evaluation by a psychiatrist or other healthcare professional with an interest in the syndrome.

6.4 **Management**

Whether or not medication is to be prescribed, behavioural management of the manifestations of ADHD will be necessary. Indeed, when symptoms are at the milder end of the spectrum, behavioural approaches will be the mainstay of interventions. Behavioural techniques require a consistency of approach and mean working with parents, carers, school staff, and others.

In a sporting context, whilst the coach may be pivotal in implementing behavioural strategies, all those working with the athlete will need to understand what approach is being taken and why.

Without a behavioural endoskeleton, those with ADHD require the external structure of an exoskeleton. Someone else has to supplement the executive functions of the frontal lobes (the 'human'). For anyone working with athletes with ADHD, emotional intelligence and structured routine is likely to be crucial. The athlete/player will then engage with the sport without inhibition or fear.

In principle, what is required is to avoid criticism. This will 'lose' the person as those with ADHD will have been experiencing criticism from authority figures since childhood. Simplicity and clarity, with instructions that are concrete, rehearsed, and brief, are recommended. This is followed by checks that the athlete has understood what has been asked. This step is crucial. Emphasize routine and avoid unexpected changes. If change is required, it should be signalled clearly and simply in advance.

If a player becomes angry, investigate the preceding sequence. It may be that the athlete misunderstood what was said, misinterpreted the intent, or felt provoked.

Tips for managing suspected ADHD include the following:

• Avoid anger or irritation; surprise by praise
• Use short sentences with one idea at a time
• Ensure the player does really understand instructions, and is not just pretending to (best achieved through 1:1 dialogue)
• Use visual material as well as words
• Avoid unexpected change.

Techniques that simplify the task enable sustained focus. This might include learning to repeat a simple phrase when needed such as 'Your job is just to … '. Visual memory is often more intact than verbal memory so visual material and diagrams may be especially important. Payne Stewart, a professional golfer reported to have had ADHD, won the 1999 US Open using techniques developed with his psychologist. Before each shot he was reminded to identify an intermediate target (a visual cue) prior to hitting the ball.

Case study

A talented footballer was often in conflict with other players and coaches. Although her technical skills and ball control were superb (making her extremely popular with fans), she did not follow her coach's instructions on the pitch. This led to frustration in the dug-out, confrontations with the coaching staff, and increasingly angry defiance from the player.

She changed clubs and a new coach intuitively understood that she was troubled rather than simply wilful. The new coach worked with her in 1:1 sessions and made it clear that she was appreciated, and perhaps even a victim of injustice (empathizing with the player's view). Her coach worked on explaining exactly what was wanted on the pitch and supplemented this with diagrams. To begin with she would nod her agreement but when probed had clearly not fully grasped what was required. The coach eventually learned how to express ideas clearly and more simply and then to check her understanding at each stage. Conflicts would still occur from time to time but were less frequent and the player knew she would get a fair hearing. The partnership prospered and she became a valuable asset to the team.

6.5 Drug treatments

Medication is often used to help people with ADHD self-manage the complexities of our culture and the environment around them (Table 6.1). Methylphenidate remains the mainstay of these treatments, especially when symptoms are moderate to severe. It appears to work by 'switching on' the frontal cortex (via increased extracellular dopamine in related neural tracts) and this helps to compensate for the deficits in executive function associated with these brain areas. For some, the effect is dramatic; irritable, restless children become capable of conversations and can concentrate to study.

One important consequence when treating a medical ailment in an athlete is that this helps to 'level the playing field'. It allows a player to compete with his/her peers without disadvantage. In a sporting context, prescribed stimulants may help a player to track the game and play in a more strategic manner and compensate for some of the deficits found in these areas in ADHD sufferers.

Methylphenidate is a powerful stimulant and along with other therapeutic and illicit stimulants is banned for use in competitive sportspeople for this reason (see Chapter 9). Achieving 'a level playing field' requires that prescribed medication is not performance enhancement by another route. The issue of stimulant misuse is addressed if stimulant medication is only authorized and used after the kind of robust specialist evaluation described in Section 6.2.

When treated, some adolescents report losing spontaneity, becoming too serious (or inhibited) to bond with their teammates, and too thoughtful to react quickly on the field of play. A side effect of stimulants is also to suppress appetite—a problem for sports where calorie intake or muscle bulk is important. These issues need careful consideration. Side effects that are detrimental to sports performance will limit the use of good treatments if it means that athletes are less willing to take them.

Issues of tolerability and side effects can be partially addressed by using short-acting agents such as methylphenidate. Short-acting drugs may improve social and academic performance and help with otherwise challenging areas: paying bills, organizing children, driving, and any complex tasks involving planning, concentration, and organization. They can be used to assist in daily life but without compromising performance on the field of play. Atomoxetine is not a banned drug and may offer an alternative although it too can have an effect on appetite. It is not effective when taken intermittently and

Table 6.1 Drugs used in the treatment of ADHD

Drug	Category (duration of action)	WADA prohibition	Notes
Methylphenidate	Short-acting stimulant (3–6 hours or 12 hours for extended-release formulation)	Competition only (TUE required)	Monitor pulse, blood pressure (BP), weight (and height if still growing) at least 6-monthly
Dexamfetamine	Short-acting stimulant (3–6 hours). Used in refractory ADHD	Competition only (TUE required)	Monitor pulse, BP, weight (and height if still growing) at least 6-monthly
Lisdexamfetamine	Longer-acting stimulant (6–8 hours). Pro-drug of dexamfetamine. Used in refractory ADHD	Competition only (TUE required)	Monitor pulse, BP, weight (and height if still growing) at least 6-monthly
Atomoxetine	Long-acting, non-stimulant noradrenergic reuptake inhibitor (24 hours)	No	Not first line in many countries so there is no WADA requirement to trial this first before granting TUE
Modafinil	Stimulant	Competition only (TUE required)	Used for narcolepsy. Unlicensed in ADHD (case reports of Stevens–Johnson syndrome)
Bupropion	Antidepressant, although unlicensed in some countries, and stimulant (variable half-life of 3–16 hours)	No (under review)	Also used for smoking cessation. Unlicensed in ADHD. Risk of seizures at higher doses

variable dosing regimens are not appropriate as a way of managing side effects that may impair performance.

As well as being performance enhancing, stimulants can be harmful. Earlier concerns that stimulant use would promote increased violence from users on the sports field have proved unfounded. In general, ADHD sufferers are less violent when taking appropriate medication. However, dopamine affects brain reward mechanisms and stimulants seem to delay or override signals to stop exercising. Amphetamine use to enhance performance in endurance events such as road cyclists has been associated with potentially fatal hyperthermia and may have contributed to the high-profile death of British cyclist Tom Simpson in the 1967 Tour de France. It is the duty of all doctors to 'do no harm' and prescribed drugs should not create unacceptable risk to health when used in the sports arena.

6.6 Conclusion

The right sport may provide an environment where a person who has struggled with ADHD can excel, without medication or therapy, where some of the characteristics of ADHD may not necessarily create a disadvantage. Those coaching young people are likely to encounter ADHD. It is a common condition, affects adults as well as children and adolescents, and is not a barrier to sports participation even at the highest levels. Affected individuals are not non-compliant, deliberately defiant, or wilful trouble-makers. They may be unintentionally blunt and it may simply be that they do not understand what is being asked and require more routine than some others. It is important to spot this and not to fall into the trap of all the other adults in their lives by become angry or dismissive. The coach needs to be 'the human' to help the athlete cope with their 'chimp'. Finally, medical interventions are available and can be adapted to be acceptable, tolerable, and safe in the sporting arena.

Further reading

Angold, A. and Costello, E.J. (2000). The Child and Adolescent Psychiatric Assessment (CAPA). *J Am Acad Child Adolesc Psychiatry* 39:39–48.

Asherson, P., Chen, W., Craddock, B., and Taylor, E. (2007). Adult attention deficit hyperactivity disorder: recognition and treatment in general adult psychiatry *Br J Psychiatry* 190:4–5.

Bolea-Alamanac, B., Nutt, D., Adamou, M., Asherson, P., Bazire, S., Coghill, D., *et al.* (2014). Evidence based guidelines for the pharmacological management of ADHD: update on recommendations from the British Association for Pharmacology. *J Psychopharmacol* 28:179–203.

McArdle, P. (2004). ADHD and life span development. *Br J Psychiatry* 184:468–469.

Brown, T.E. (2013). *A New Understanding of ADHD in Children and Adults.* New York: Routledge.

Chapter 7

The athletic personality and personality disorders

Bruce Owen

Key points

- No single personality type distinguishes athletes from non-athletes.
- A number of personality traits have been shown to occur more commonly in athletes including extraversion, perfectionism, and conscientiousness.
- Personality traits can be functional and have been associated with high-level sports performance.
- Personality disorders occur in athletes and can have a significant impact on their functioning, particularly when managing stress and interpersonal relationships.
- Athletic identity, a measure of how much an athlete's involvement in sport defines their identity, can be both functional and dysfunctional for an athlete's performance and broader life.

7.1 Introduction

Although the term personality is familiar to most people it is helpful to consider its characteristics and what defines it. Personality describes the patterns of thinking, feeling, and acting that constitute a person's response to life situations. It is considered to be present from late adolescence, stable over time, and consistent across different environments.

Different approaches have been taken to describe or classify normal personality differences, the oldest being to group people into distinct types. Early models included Sheldon's work which theorized three personality types based on physique:

- Endomporphs—physically round and tend to be sociable, fun loving, and relaxed
- Ectomorphs—physically thinner and characterized by being self-conscious, shy, and private
- Mesomorphs—described as more muscular and typically confident, courageous, and competitive.

Whilst this was an interesting theory, it was lacking in any evidence. A model based on three types or categories does not work well when describing the complex nature of personality. As understanding has improved, a trait approach is now favoured.

The trait approach is based on breaking down personality into dimensions and then assessing an individual in each of these dimensions to determine their profile. This works on the basis that there are universal dimensions that can be measured in everyone.

For most people, their personality allows them to interact with others and function well. This is not always the case and there are times when personality traits can be unhelpful. When an individual's personality traits have an adverse impact on aspects of their functioning, resulting in disadvantage and distress for them and others, the term personality disorder is used. Managing interpersonal and social relationships and managing emotions and feelings are areas that people with personality disorders might find particularly difficult.

There has been much interest in the theory that athletes may differ from non-athletes in personality profile, and that the personality of athletes differs in different sports, and there is some evidence in support of this.

It is important for those working with athletes to have an understanding of how an athlete's personality type may be functional, for both their performance and general functioning, but also at times dysfunctional. Having this understanding helps those working with athletes to support them more effectively.

7.2 Assessment of personality

Most methods of assessment of personality describe characteristics in quantitative terms. The most widely used tests are self-completed inventories that ask individuals about themselves and their beliefs and attitudes. There are a variety of such tests and each produces slightly different information. All tests have in common that they provide a profile of a person made up of scores on each of several aspects of personality—usually called personality dimensions.

It is important to be aware of the difference between personality types and dimensions. Dimensions relate to areas of personality that are important in interactions. One example of a dimension is extroversion where each individual will be within a range with highly extrovert behaviours (very outgoing, enthusiastic, and sociable) at one end of a continuum and low levels of extroversion (quiet and more reserved) at the other. An individual's personality type describes the combination of dimensions. Many dimensions have been described and measured but five in particular have gained prominence. These are sometimes known as the 'big five' (Table 7.1).

An assessment of personality can also be made by a clinical interview or series of interviews. This may be a structured interview using an assessment tool or form part of a more general psychiatric or psychological assessment. In practice, a clinician working with an athlete may assess personality over a period of time using a more qualitative approach. In this way, rather than basing the assessment on scores from assessment tools, it is based on the history of the individual and how they have behaved over time in a range of environments including personal and work life. How an individual has managed relationships and stresses or conflict is particularly important in an assessment like this.

Table 7.1 Description of the 'big five' personality dimensions

Personality dimension	High-scorer description	Low-scorer description
Extroversion	Outgoing, sociable, assertive, excitement seeking	Quiet, reserved, cautious
Conscientiousness	Organized, systematic, achievement orientated	Spontaneous, disorganized, easily distracted
Agreeableness	Trusting, even tempered, tolerant, sensitive	Suspicious, critical, ruthless
Neuroticism	Anxious, irritable, prone to worry and negative emotions	Calm, emotionally stable, risk takers
Openness	Open to new ideas, curious, creative, and imaginative	Practical, rational, sceptical, and pragmatic

7.3 **Personality traits in athletes**

There has been considerable interest and research in the links between sport and personality traits. No particular personality type or profile that distinguishes athletes from non-athletes has been identified. This is likely to reflect both the wide range of sports studied and dimensions measured. There have, however, across a range of sports, been some consistent observations in relation to certain dimensions. Athletes have been found to have higher scores on the measure of conscientiousness and indeed in some studies this has been associated with performance consistency and longevity. This characteristic also predicts success in a range of non-sporting vocations.

Two of the other big five characteristics appear to differ in athletes when compared to non-athletes, again across a range of sports. Athletes tend to score more highly for extroversion and have lower scores for neuroticism suggesting greater emotional stability. Interestingly there is some evidence this latter characteristic may be associated with performance in a high level of competitive stress. Perfectionism and anger also have particular significance in sport and are discussed in more detail in Section 7.3.1.

There have been studies looking at how personality characteristics vary between team and individual sports. The findings have face validity, with there being some evidence of athletes in team sports tending to score comparatively higher on the measure of agreeableness and sociotropy (a measure of how much an individual provides support and depends on others) and athletes in individual sports scoring higher in autonomy as well as conscientiousness.

In many areas of life, personality attributes are used to try and predict success. An example of this is their use in the selection processes within a range of professions. In sport this is relatively new. There is emerging evidence, however, that personality attributes could be used along with other measures to predict success—an interesting area that may become more important with further research.

7.3.1 **Perfectionism**

Perfectionism relates to thoughts, expectations, and how events are interpreted. An individual with perfectionist traits will:

- set and then compulsively pursue excessively high goals
- be overly self-critical in evaluating achievements.

It is recognized that athletes often have perfectionist traits although the consequences of this are not always clear. There is some evidence that perfectionism may be a helpful trait associated with improved performance. However, there is also significant evidence that it can lead to performance hindering anxiety, burn out, and an increased risk of depression and eating disorders. This is especially the case when the self-critical element of perfectionism is pronounced.

It is suggested that the origin of perfectionism may be an important factor. The simplest models look at two types:

- Normal, positive, or adaptive perfectionism where there is a positive drive to achievement
- Unhealthy, negative, or maladaptive perfectionism where the drive comes from a fear of failure.

There is a link between self-esteem and positive perfectionism, suggesting this form of perfectionism may confer some benefit. However, the negative type is more often associated with anxiety.

Perfectionism has also been described as having three dimensions:

- Self-orientated—excessively high standards of own performance
- Other-orientated—excessively high standards of another
- Socially prescribed—perceiving others to hold excessively high standards of you.

Studying the effect of perfectionism using this model suggests that self-orientated perfectionism does not have the negative associations with burnout found in the other two. Socially prescribed perfectionism (perhaps related to parents or coaches) has also been associated with the development of low mood in athletes.

There is an association between parental perfectionism (the athlete's assessment of this) and athlete perfectionism. It is important to be aware of the role parents and coaches can have in the development and maintenance of perfectionism in athletes. Awareness of factors that may be contributing to this can help parents and coaches guard against setting unrealistic goals and defining self-worth exclusively according to achievement in sport. As well as setting unrealistic goals and under-rating achievements, individuals who are perfectionist may also be at risk of overtraining. These factors need to be considered in supporting athletes with goal setting, training programmes, and a realistic and helpful assessment of their achievements.

Case study 1

Richard is a young, male, elite middle distance runner who sustained a soft tissue injury to his ankle during competition 3 months previously. His recovery has been delayed and the team physiotherapist has referred him for advice thinking he may be becoming distressed by the impact on his training and performance.

A full psychiatric history reveals that concern about the impact of his injury on his performance is beginning to lead to Richard feeling low in mood and to experience anxiety about his future. It is apparent that he feels he is letting down not just himself but also his coach and parents. He acknowledges that the level of anxiety has led him to return to training earlier than recommended. He has also stated that he tends to add in additional sessions to those recommended by his coach.

Richard was helped by his physiotherapist to look at the impact of overtraining. He was also supported in setting short-term goals that helped him adhere to a more gradual build-up of training over time consistent with his injury recovery. Key to this was getting his consent to work with his coach and parents to plan his training programme and set goals.

7.3.2 **Anger and aggression**

Aggression is generally a desirable trait within sport. It can manifest in different ways through risk-taking behaviour, an aggressive approach to the rules, and physical aggression in contact sports. All of these can offer a competitive advantage but can become counterproductive leading to a loss of control or rule breaking that results in penalties and may lose a match. It is when aggression is counterproductive that it is likely to come to clinical attention.

When an athlete presents with problems with anger or aggression it is helpful to take a biopsychosocial approach to determine factors contributing to this—treatment or management of these being the primary goal. This holistic approach to assessment and management is integral to contemporary psychiatric practice recognizing that biological, psychological, and social factors must be considered in assessment and formulation. The approach is based on the principle that no one patient or health condition can be reduced to a single aspect and that the three domains are relevant. Key when making the assessment is collecting a thorough history of the problem. This includes whether it is a longstanding problem or a new development and noting any recent changes in the form of biological or psychosocial stresses.

Biological

There are a number of biological factors that can lead to increased aggression. Rarely, it is secondary to an underlying physical illness resulting in changes in hormonal levels including testosterone or oestrogen. More commonly, athletes taking substances either to enhance performance, for recreational reasons, or medical reasons may, as a secondary effect, develop increased aggression. Examples would include use of anabolic steroids, stimulants, or alcohol (which can contribute to aggression both during intoxication and between drinking bouts). Underlying mental illness should also be considered with mood disorders (both depression and bipolar disorder) and attention deficit hyperactivity disorder being associated with aggression.

Psychological

Psychological factors can contribute to problems with control of aggression. A parent's response to a child who is behaving aggressively will influence how they learn to control their aggression. Control of emotions develops during childhood and adolescence. In some individuals who develop personality disorders this control is not achieved, resulting in an increased risk of impulsive and aggressive behaviour. These problems are particularly associated with what are known as cluster B personality disorders (described in more detail in Section 7.5). Acute psychological stresses can also be factors that increase anger and aggression and identifying these stresses is important in the initial assessment.

Social

Social factors are relevant in the development of aggression and its modulation. The environment an athlete experienced as a child as well as in their current setting will influence their perception of what is socially normal behaviour. Sport can provide the boundaries to help athletes develop control of aggression and other emotions. If, however, the environment promotes aggression, for example, if it is modelled through others, then this can result in increased levels of aggressive behaviour.

A thorough assessment will inform how the problem is to be managed. Some factors may need to be addressed first in order to allow psychological treatments to begin (e.g. problems with alcohol, substance misuse, or immediate social stressors). Psychological approaches most commonly used include cognitive behavioural therapy, relaxation therapy, and social skills training, each delivered over a time-limited period, usually around eight to ten sessions.

7.4 **Athletic identity**

Identity refers to how someone perceives themselves, including elements of their personality. It has been said to be what connects the individual with society. Many people have a number of different roles in their lives (such as family, academic, or work roles) and these form components of their identity.

The term athletic identity refers to the degree that an athlete identifies with their athletic role and looks to others for acknowledgement of that role. For some athletes, particularly elite athletes, the amount of time, physical and psychological energy dedicated to sport can mean that other aspects of their life become secondary and neglected and the athletic identity dominates.

In assessing athletic identity three factors are important:

- Social identity—the degree to which someone sees themselves as occupying the role of an athlete

- Exclusivity—a measure of the degree to which self-worth is dependent on athletic role

- Negative affectivity—the extent to which negative sporting outcomes result in negative emotions.

Having a strong athletic identity can confer advantages, for example, a strong athletic identity correlates with more frequent physical activity and thus greater fitness levels. It has also been found to offer wider benefits including more confident social interactions, greater commitment to sport, and, in some studies, higher levels of performance.

However, a strong athletic identity does create risks for an athlete and it is the exclusivity factor of athletic identity that carries a particular risk. These risks can be present both during an athlete's competitive career and afterwards. Whilst an athlete is competing, a strong athletic identity can lead to maladaptive acts such as overtraining. There is a particular risk of this during injury when reduced training can lead to anxiety, loss of confidence, and depression. A strong athletic identity is also thought to contribute to the use of performance-enhancing drugs.

Arguably the greatest risk occurs when an athlete ceases to compete, either due to injury or retirement. Where an athlete's self-worth is strongly linked to their sporting role the loss of this role can be a very difficult adjustment and associated with a delay in future career development, physical, and psychological health problems. There is evidence that this may be a particular problem for athletes in sports where the peak of performance is early and where there is an exclusive focus on sport from a young age (such as female gymnastics). For all athletes, having interests outside of sport would appear to reduce these risks. Sporting organizations should aim to support athletes to find the optimum position between a life exclusively devoted to sport and a life where outside interests are a distraction that limits achievement.

Case study 2

Mike is a 19-year-old and was scouted at the age of 9 to join the youth academy of a top-flight football team. He performed well through his mid-teens and remained in the academy. He signed a professional contract at the age of 17. He was loaned out to a lower league club a year ago and has only played very occasional games. His will be out of contract in 6 months.

He was referred to his general practitioner as he was noted to be low in mood, was withdrawing from his friends, and there had been frequent outbursts of anger, both whilst playing football and in other situations.

An assessment revealed that from early in his life he had focused most of his energies on his football career. He had no school qualifications and his identity was based entirely on his role as a footballer. The main elements of treatment involved working with him and his family to build other aspects of his life and to explore other roles. These had remained minor while his football career was his primary focus. He returned to education through evening classes and completed a coaching qualification. This reduced the pressure he was placing on himself to succeed in his playing career and resulted in him achieving more both in the subsequent football season and more broadly in his education and secondary career as a coach.

7.5 **Personality disorders**

In small numbers of people, personality traits have such a profound adverse impact on all aspects of their functioning that they result in significant disadvantage and distress for themselves and others. In these situations, the term personality disorder is often used. In considering such a diagnosis it is important that the personality features and related dysfunctional behaviours are evident across a range of aspects of someone's life, stable over time, and present from early adulthood.

Several types of personality disorder have been described based on the observation that there are particular patterns of personality traits. These types are commonly placed into three broad clusters reflecting common or overlapping emotional content:

- Cluster A—difficulty relating to others and can appear odd or eccentric
- Cluster B—difficulty regulating emotions and feelings, can appear dramatic, emotional, and volatile
- Cluster C—experience overwhelming fear and anxiety.

Table 7.2 Types of personality disorder			
Cluster A	*Paranoid*: sensitive to criticism, tendency to bear grudges, suspicious, excessive self-importance, preoccupied with conspiratorial explanations	*Schizoid*: emotionally detached, limited capacity to express warmth or emotion, solitary lifestyle, indifference to views of others, preoccupied with fantasy	*Schizotypal*: odd or eccentric behaviour and beliefs, limited emotional expression, poor rapport with others, suspicious	
Cluster B	*Emotionally unstable*: Impulsive nature, emotionally volatile, feel empty, intense relationships and excessive efforts to avoid abandonment, use of self-harm as coping strategy	*Antisocial*: lack of concern for others, disregard rules, low tolerance to frustration, show aggression and violence with no feelings of guilt or responsibility	*Histrionic*: exaggerated expression of emotion, self-centred, suggestible, labile affect, and over-concern with physical appearance	*Narcissistic*: self-important, crave attention, imagine great success for self, take advantage of others
Cluster C	*Anxious*: feel anxious and tense most of the time, low self-esteem, avoid a range of social and occupational situations due to fear of criticism	*Anankastic*: feelings of doubt and caution, preoccupation with rules and order, rigid and pedantic, unreasonable expectation that others will do as they expect	*Dependant*: passive, reluctant to make demands on others, encourage others to make decisions for them, fear of being alone	

Within each cluster there are a number of separate personality disorder types (Table 7.2). Although many people fit neatly into one particular category, others have characteristics that fit with more than one categorization or overlap with several types.

Key features of a personality disorder are that it develops in early life, persists over time, and impacts across all or most areas of life. As with most health problems there can be a considerable range in the severity of personality disorders. They can, and often do, fluctuate in severity, largely dependent on the stresses and supports around an individual at any one time. The difficulties may only become apparent to others when either stresses increase or supports reduce. This results in an exaggeration of the emotions experienced and subsequent dysfunctional behaviours. During assessment it usually becomes quickly apparent that the key features have always been present albeit at times in an attenuated form.

There is little work looking at the prevalence of personality disorders in athletes. Where this has been studied it appears that the range of personality disorders is present although some specific personality disorders (anankastic or obsessive, narcissistic, and emotionally unstable) occur more frequently in athletes.

How an individual responds under stress is particularly important. Stress is inherent to competitive sport and effective techniques to manage this are needed. Clinicians working with athletes with a personality disorder will find it useful to understand how the athlete respond to stresses, their motivating drives, and which are their most adaptive techniques for dealing with the stressors that can be anticipated in the sporting arena.

7.6 **Working with people with personality disorders**

Possibly the most important factor in working with someone who has a personality disorder is to understand both the problem and how it impacts across a range of commonly encountered situations. This allows the athlete/patient and clinician to agree on appropriate levels of support as well as the nature of that support and reduces the likelihood of problems escalating.

7.6.1 **Psychological treatments**

Specific psychological treatments have been found to be helpful for people with personality disorders. These vary considerably in their duration and are most widely used in people with cluster B personality disorders. These are the disorders that most frequently present to health services.

* Dialectical behaviour therapy—based on cognitive behavioural therapy but adapted to help people who experience emotions more intensely. In this form of therapy the relationship with the therapist is particularly important. Therapy usually involves both individual sessions and skills training in groups. It is typically offered over a 1-year period.

* Cognitive behavioural therapy—focuses on the link between thoughts and feelings and is a way to change unhelpful patterns of thinking. This widely available treatment can be offered as individual or group therapy. It typically involves up to 20 weekly or fortnightly sessions.

* Cognitive analytical therapy—the focus here is on helping to identify and adapt unhelpful patterns of behaviour, particularly in relationships. It is an individual therapy and typically involves weekly sessions for 8–24 weeks.

* Dynamic psychotherapy—a longer-term therapy, usually lasting a year or more, that helps people explore and understand the impact of past experiences on their current emotions and behaviours.

* Interpersonal therapy—focuses on relationships and the impact these have on mental health. A relatively brief therapy typically of 8–16 sessions.

7.6.2 **Medication**

Whilst medication is not the mainstay of treatment for any personality disorder it can be helpful in reducing some of the associated symptoms. Antidepressants can help with the low mood often present in cluster B personality disorders and can also help reduce anxiety. Some antidepressants and mood stabilizing medication (e.g. sodium valproate, lamotrigine, and lithium) can be useful in reducing impulsivity and aggression but are not licensed for this purpose and should only be prescribed under specialist supervision.

Case study 3

MS is a 20-year-old gymnast who competes at an elite level. She was a member of the national squad and was recovering from an injury in the lead up to a major meeting. She was included in the team to travel to the meeting but informed on arriving that she would not be competing in her preferred individual event although she would be included in the team event. MS did not attend the pre-meeting training session and was found to have stayed in her hotel room and refused to come out. After lengthy discussions with her coach through a closed door she informed the team she had taken an overdose of paracetamol the evening before.

At this point the team management sought psychiatric help. Through discussions with her and the team it was apparent that she had felt an overwhelming sense of rejection at not being selected to compete in her preferred event. She thought that her coach, who she had previously found to be very supportive, had lost faith in her and that there was no hope for her in the future.

MS has an emotionally unstable personality disorder and looking back it was evident that although she had never had such a severe reaction to stress before, she had been volatile and come into conflict with a number of the squad previously. Her relationship with her coach had been more intense than the usual gymnast/coach relationship.

She was helped considerably by psychological therapy. The focus of the therapy was in helping her recognize how she felt and reacted at times of stress, developing coping strategies to manage this, and building her self-esteem. The coaching team were able to get support for themselves to support her and help her to manage her stresses. This included ensuring psychological support was available when needed and predictably at times of stress. It was also helpful to clarify the roles and boundaries of the coaching relationship and adopt a clearer approach to communication.

Further reading

Burton, R.W. (2005). Aggression in sport. In Tofler, I.R. and Morse, E.D. (Eds.), *Clinics in Sports Medicine: The Interface between Sport Psychiatry & Sports Medicine* (pp. 845–52). Philadelphia, PA: Elsevier Saunders.

Chamorro-Premuzic, T. (2007). *Personality and Individual Differences*. Chichester: Wiley.

Evershed, S. (2011). Treatment of personality disorder: skills-based therapies. *Adv Psychiatr Treat* 17:206–13.

Hendawy, H.M.F.M. and Awad, E.A.A. (2013). Personality and personality disorders in athletes. In Baron, D.A., Reardon, C.L., and Baron, S.H. (Eds.), *Clinical Sports Psychiatry: An international Perspective* (pp. 53–64). Chichester: Wiley-Blackwell.

Murphy, S.M. (2012). *The Oxford Handbook of Sport and Exercise Psychology*. New York: Oxford University Press.

Peters, S. (2012). *The Chimp Paradox: The Mind Management Programme to Help You Achieve Success, Confidence and Happiness*. London: Vermillion.

Tyrer, P., Coombs, N., Ibrahimi, F., Mathilakath, A., Bajaj, P., Ranger, M., *et al.* (2007). Critical developments in the assessment of personality disorder. *Br J Psychiatry* 190(Suppl. 49):s51–s59.

Chapter 8

Exercise participation and mental health

Alan Currie and Reshad Malik

Key points

- Physical activity improves emotional well-being including symptoms of anxiety and depression and cognitive function.
- Poor physical health is significantly associated with a range of psychiatric conditions and could be improved by physical activity.
- Sport and exercise participation can support social inclusion and recovery in chronic severe mental illness.

8.1 Introduction

As this chapter discusses the impact of exercise on mental health, it is important to make the distinction between physical activity, exercise, and sport. Caspersen and colleagues (1985) describe physical activity as 'any bodily movement produced by skeletal muscles that results in energy expenditure' and exercise as 'planned, structured and repetitive bodily movement, the objective of which is to improve or maintain physical fitness'. According to these definitions, you can be physically active without technically engaging in exercise. The *Oxford English Dictionary* defines sport as any activity involving physical exertion and skill in which an individual or team competes against others for entertainment.

8.2 Exercise and mental health

Across all age ranges, exercise has been found to improve aspects of mental health. For example, exercise enhances general emotional well-being, leads to a reduction in depressive symptoms, and can protect against depressive relapses. Resistance training reduces subjective feelings of anger and tension and twin studies have shown a correlation between leg strength and higher objective measures of cognition.

In older adults, exercise can act as a buffer for age-related cognitive decline. The physical health benefits of regular exercise may confer an indirect and secondary benefit in cognition whilst reducing blood pressure, for example, can lower the risk of cardiovascular or cerebrovascular events that may precipitate cognitive decline. Direct mechanisms by which exercise has been postulated to prevent cognitive decline include enhanced synaptic plasticity, anti-amyloid effects, and enhancement of executive function (see also Section 8.3.1).

Many studies on the impact of exercise on mental health consider its role in the treatment of depressive disorders where it has been advocated as an adjunct to usual treatment. A review in 2009 identified 25 randomized trials comparing exercise with either no treatment or an established treatment (e.g. talking therapy) for depressive disorders. Exercise improved the symptoms of depression, although it was not possible to determine the most effective type of exercise. Evidence suggests that exercise may need to be sustained for a significant period for benefits on mood to be maintained.

The relationship between exercise and mental health is circular; for example, low mood or high levels of anxiety can lead to decreased activity either through lack of motivation or as safety behaviour. Reduced motivation and activity lowers mood by multiple routes. These include fewer and less stimulating social contacts, fewer opportunities for pleasurable experiences, and absence of the beneficial neuroendocrine response to physical activity. Safety behaviours usually involve some means of avoiding an anxiety-provoking situation. They provide temporary relief but are an obstacle to overcoming the source of anxiety in the longer term. Safety behaviours may even escalate the irrational fears attached to the situation that is being avoided and in this way exacerbate anxiety levels. It is important to consider these cycles when promoting exercise as a treatment and explaining this to a patient provides a useful context and rationale for introducing exercise as an intervention.

8.3 **Exercise and physical health**

Poor fitness levels are a significant predictor of many poor health outcomes and a sedentary lifestyle is associated with less good physical and mental health. Conversely, public physical activity programmes can confer a cost-effective reduction in disease risk over a lifetime and sustained, vigorous physical activity is associated with improved survival and healthy ageing in older men.

8.3.1 **Metabolic syndrome**

Metabolic syndrome is a collection of clinical signs and abnormal laboratory findings recognized by the World Health Organization as a major, worldwide public health problem. It is associated with a threefold increase in heart attack and stroke risk. The syndrome is two to three times more prevalent in the severely mentally ill. In schizophrenia, the prevalence is five times the population level with women especially at risk and up to a third of depressed patients may have features of the syndrome.

Metabolic syndrome is multifactorial in origin and the relationship with mental illness is bidirectional. Characteristics of severe mental illness promote the development of metabolic syndrome whilst the syndrome itself increases psychiatric morbidity and especially depression.

Metabolic syndrome has five key features and a diagnosis is usually made when three of the five are present, although different authorities apply different threshold criteria for each component:

- Central adiposity: waist/hip ratio > 0.90 (men) and > 0.85 (women) or body mass index > 30 kg/m^2
- Raised blood pressure > 140/90 mmHg
- Raised triglycerides > 1.7 mmol/L
- Low high-density lipoprotein cholesterol: < 0.9 mmol/L (men) and < 1.0 mmol/L (women)
- Raised fasting glucose.

Genetics

Genetic factors are implicated. Schizophrenia is associated with an increased risk of diabetes mellitus that has a strong familial component. There are common genetic contributions to both metabolic syndrome and schizophrenia and a genetic subtype of schizophrenia patients who are more likely to gain weight.

Inflammation

Chronic inflammatory processes also contribute. Adipose tissue produces inflammatory molecules that are thought to promote insulin resistance, dyslipidaemias, and the development of atherosclerotic plaques. Metabolic syndrome is also associated with cognitive decline, perhaps via neuro-inflammation and impaired glucose metabolism. Insulin resistance is associated with the production of pro-inflammatory cytokines leading to beta-amyloid deposition (the main component of amyloid plaques found in Alzheimer's disease) and, in a vicious circle, more cytokine production.

Hypothalamic–pituitary–adrenal axis

Activation of the hypothalamic–pituitary–adrenal (HPA) axis in depression (as well as post-traumatic stress disorder and some personality disorders) can lead to a pseudo-cushingoid picture with visceral adiposity, hyperinsulinaemia, insulin resistance, hypertension, and dyslipidaemias.

Drug effects

Psychotropic drugs also have a role. The second generation of antipsychotic drugs (such as olanzapine and risperidone) is associated with more weight gain than older, first-generation drugs such as haloperidol. Several mechanisms are thought to be responsible. 5-HT$_{2C}$ receptor antagonism reduces the uptake of glucose by skeletal muscle and increases insulin resistance whilst histaminergic antagonism slows metabolism and increases sedation. Tricyclic antidepressants such as amitriptyline are also antagonistic at histamine receptors and selective serotonin re-uptake inhibiting antidepressants are associated with weight gain during long-term use.

Lifestyle

Lifestyle factors make a direct (and modifiable) contribution to the development of metabolic syndrome. Chronic psychosis, especially when negative symptoms such as amotivation, social withdrawal, and affective blunting are present, is associated with poor diet, smoking, and an inactive, impoverished daily life. A sedentary lifestyle will also reduce serotonin synthesis, promoting and exacerbating depressive symptoms.

8.3.2 **Exercise and physical activity in metabolic syndrome**

The management of metabolic syndrome includes adequate treatment of any underlying mental illness with careful attention to choice of drug especially if long-term use is anticipated. Alongside this are a series of targeted interventions that include offering help with smoking cessation and problem drinking and treating disordered glucose metabolism, dyslipidaemias, and hypertension in the standard manner.

For those with metabolic syndrome in association with a mental illness, there will be a number of factors to be addressed but for many, physical activity could have a central role. Physical activity reduces adiposity, has a positive effect on the HPA axis, is a useful intervention in negative symptoms, and can support the lifestyle changes necessary to reduce risk.

Weight management is a major challenge but central to addressing the syndrome. Actively involving those with long-term psychiatric conditions in structured exercise programmes and/or recreational sport has many potential benefits and few, if any, harmful consequences. For many it is easier to manage weight by increasing energy expenditure than by reducing intake and it is clearly advantageous to do both. Activities that are pleasurable and supported by peers (such as sport and communal exercise) are more likely to be sustained. Exercise is a means to manage stress and the related HPA axis dysregulation that is associated with the syndrome. Participation in exercise and sport also provides a means of improving social skills and receiving peer support with lifestyle changes.

Whilst physical activity may begin within mental health services (on inpatient wards and within community teams), for these interventions to be effective and sustained then partnerships within the wider community are needed. As recovery progresses, a patient may move from highly structured activities on a ward to supported activities within a community team and ultimately to independent physical activity in a local leisure facility. Good relations and communication between mental health services and leisure facilities are invaluable in allowing progress along this pathway.

8.4 **Recovery and chronic ill health**

8.4.1 **Recovery definitions**

The commonest usage of the term 'recovery' is to describe the experience of being cured of an ailment spontaneously or by an intervention or treatment. The illness or disease is removed and the patient restored to full health once more. This model fits very well with many acute conditions such as an infection treated with antibiotics or an acute musculoskeletal injury.

'Recovery' has been used in a different manner when describing the experience of those who suffer from chronic conditions where cure and full restoration of health and function is considered unattainable. Here the aim of treatment may be to minimize the impact of the illness, to support adjustment (both psychological and physical) to the limitations caused by the illness, and to accommodate these limitations into daily life. The life experience of someone with a chronic illness who is 'in recovery' is not just optimal treatment and symptom control but also 'a satisfying, hopeful and contributing life even with the limitations caused by illness'.

Individuals who are experiencing recovery will be those who have found (or been helped to find) new ways to participate and new ways to fulfil valued roles in spite of illness-related limitations. Those who are socially excluded will find this adjustment harder to achieve and thus social inclusion is an important component of recovery. Among the many benefits of sports participation is its ability to promote social inclusion and thus to support recovery.

8.4.2 **Recovery practice**

There are four important elements for practitioners who are working towards recovery with those who experience chronic ill health.

Hope

With good treatment the outcome of many psychiatric conditions (e.g. psychotic illnesses) is better than many realize. In addition, optimistic health professionals have higher recovery rates and better outcomes. In the face of stigma and misunderstanding, the health professional may be a vital source of optimistic encouragement in the journey to recovery. Helping someone to find new hope in the face of their illness can include supporting them towards the increased social interactions and improved confidence that exercise and recreational sport can bring.

Identity

Re-establishing a positive identity (and one that incorporates a chronic illness) is a difficult challenge made harder by the experience of stigma and exclusion. Those who are excluded may feel that they deserve this, especially if it is a recurring and widespread experience (the phenomenon of 'self-stigma'). Those who are excluded may start to see themselves as incapable and worthless because this fits with the stereotype and how they are treated by others. Lowering of self-esteem and self-efficacy has a negative impact on sociability and confidence and this creates a barrier to participating in group sport and exercise. With support from mental health professionals, physical activity, exercise, and sport can be an important means to challenge the incapable stereotype, to begin to feel valued by others, and in turn to value oneself.

Building a life

Helping someone to move out of a dependent and disability-enhancing sick role is a major rehabilitative challenge. This is achieved by setting appropriate goals that help an individual to move away from a dependent sick role and ultimately away from healthcare services towards full independence. All kinds of activities (including sports) can be useful in this process and can be introduced gradually with an appropriate (and perhaps diminishing) level of healthcare support at each stage. A graded approach might begin with a highly structured activity exclusively in a healthcare setting, before progressing to providing support to access mainstream sports/exercise facilities, and ultimately to completely independent use.

Efficacy

Feeling able to control symptoms and how they impact on daily life is a key component in adjusting to the limitations an illness may impose. Having the skills and confidence to manage symptoms is an important mediator of better functional outcomes in severe and enduring mental illness. Self-efficacy in symptom management can be achieved through specific psychological therapies (e.g. cognitive and behavioural treatment approaches) and is enhanced by exercise and sports participation. Exercise, for example, may be a useful way of reducing anxiety and stress and of achieving a state of mindfulness that improves general well-being. Sport and exercise may also be an important distraction from symptoms and problems. Individuals who are engaged in rewarding, satisfying, and social activities will also experience an enhanced sense of efficacy in managing their daily lives.

8.5 **Social inclusion and sport**

8.5.1 **Social exclusion**

Social isolation is intrinsically linked to poor mental health, which supports the idea that we are inherently social creatures. Humans have evolved as social beings. Evolution has conferred the skill of good communication as a survival advantage; firstly by the interpretation of signals and then by the development of language. This starts at birth, with neonates communicating their needs initially through crying and gradually through learning cues, expressions, signs, and language.

Loneliness consequent upon social isolation can occasionally be seen as advantageous as it is a reminder to seek the company of others to fulfil basic needs. However, when loneliness becomes persistent this has a lasting negative effect on the ability to relate and interact with others.

Social exclusion is a term in common use that describes non-participation in the activities that are central to normal day-to-day life. Those affected are excluded from employment, education, relationships, leisure activities, and much else that bring meaning and purpose to life. Being excluded can be both a cause and a consequence of mental health problems and it is not surprising that social exclusion is strongly associated with poor mental health.

Exclusions are often multiple and cumulative. For example, exclusion from employment reduces other social opportunities and enhances material poverty. Conversely, being included in one activity creates new opportunities; for example, taking up a new hobby enhances relationships and contributes to enhanced confidence and self-esteem that can then create additional opportunities.

Those with mental health problems may encounter additional stigmatizing attitudes, beliefs, and behaviours in the sports setting that are over and above their normal day-to-day experiences of stigma. There may be concerns about a person's ability to act as a team player and to support other members of the team not just physically but also emotionally. There may also be concerns that including someone with a mental health problem may negatively affect the performance of teammates. The sufferer may be seen as weak, frail, and simply 'not up to it'. These factors will create obstacles to their full inclusion in sporting activities.

8.5.2 **Exercise as a vehicle for social inclusion and recovery**

There are multiple dimensions to social inclusion:

- Spatial—the closing of social distance
- Relational—a sense of belonging and acceptance by a group

- Functional—improved knowledge, skills, and understanding
- Power—a change in perceived locus of control.

This framework illustrates the ways that participation in sport and exercise contributes to the process of social inclusion by bringing people from differing social backgrounds together in a shared interest (spatial), offering a sense of belonging to a team or club (relational), providing opportunities for the development of skills (functional), and by extending social networks and increased cohesion with the community (power). Exclusion is a common adverse experience in mental illness and hampers recovery. Sport and exercise can promote social inclusion and enhance recovery.

8.6 **Barriers to sports participation**

Barriers to participation in sport affect the general population, not just those with mental health problems. These barriers include factors such as fear of failure, other contending responsibilities, the financial cost of participation, social anxiety, feeling overwhelmed by the prospect of lifestyle modifications, and general poor motivation.

Helping patients to address these issues can be the first steps to overcoming these barriers. Realistic goals are a good starting point to make the process seem less daunting and to maintain a sense of control. Realistic goals should be short term and easy to reach, so that positive feedback will slowly build confidence and self-esteem. For example, a short-term goal could include getting off the bus a stop early that can gradually extend to more complex, demanding tasks.

SMART is a useful mnemonic when considering goals:

Specific—make sure goals are clear and not ambiguous.

Measurable—this ensures you both know when a goal has been reached.

Achievable—make goals realistic and achievable.

Relevant—goals should be relevant to the person undertaking them to maintain motivation.

Time based—setting a time period within which to achieve the goal.

Taking part in exercise is not necessarily a costly pursuit. For example, in many countries there are government-backed initiatives to encourage exercise participation such as the 2012 'Let's Get Moving' campaign in the United Kingdom. This highlights many ways in which physical activity can be incorporated into daily life for little if any cost.

Counselling approaches can be used when there are specific barriers to be overcome such as time pressures or social anxiety. For those with multiple competing demands on their time it can be helpful to consider and reflect on ways of addressing this and in particular to think of simple ways to include physical activity in the daily routine. Even mild and subclinical levels of social anxiety can be a major obstacle to participation and especially in the early stages. Advice might include accompanying a friend initially or beginning with more solitary activities such as walking. More complex group sports can be introduced as confidence and fitness build.

8.7 'Prescribing' exercise

Issuing an 'exercise prescription' is already relatively commonplace, especially in primary care. Although a moderate amount of exercise for approximately 30 minutes a day in total is a standard recommendation (something equivalent to a brisk walk where it is still possible to hold a conversation), this need not be the starting point. Indeed, the initial goal may be much lower for those whose baseline fitness is very low and who may have experienced an especially severe mental illness. There are two important points to consider: any physical activity is better than none and exercise time and intensity can be gradually increased over many weeks and months.

- Consider the practicalities of exercise for the patient before prescribing and address any barriers that may prevent adherence (see Section 8.6).

- Keep an exercise and diet journal and review this regularly to monitor progress. The journal can be reviewed at routine appointments alongside a more general review of mental state. This can be helpful in correlating progress in exercise with changes in mood and affect.

- A collaborative discussion of short- and medium-term goals can foster a sense of support and also help a patient to develop control and self-efficacy.

- The journal can be used for reflective practice when goals have been achieved (How does this feel? What has been learned? How can this help to plan the next stage?). The same reflective approach is at least as important if the patient falls short of pre-set goals (What has been learned? Does the goal need to be adjusted? What extra support might be needed to reach the goal?).

When considering exercise as a management option, it is important that the plan has multidisciplinary input—nurses, occupational therapists, and physiotherapists where available will have insight into the patient's ability and motivation and can help to set goals.

There are multiple benefits to prescribing exercise: physical, psychological, and social. The choice of exercise should take this into account. While solo, aerobic exercises such as cycling or yoga have been shown to have an impact on neuronal plasticity in schizophrenia, more team-based sports might be better for social development.

Practical steps for exercise prescription in clinical settings are summarized in Box 8.1.

Case study 1: recovery and social inclusion in psychosis

A 42-year-old man was given a diagnosis of paranoid schizophrenia after he had a psychotic breakdown at the age of 26. In the first 3 years of his illness he was admitted to hospital four times. During this time he lost his job, his relationship broke up, and he moved back to live with his mother.

His illness entered a more stable phase in his 30s with reduced symptom intensity and he could agree that treatment had been helpful. He was always adherent to medication and to the monitoring regimen of blood tests. However, he had some concerns about treatment as he had gained weight and often felt sluggish.

Three years ago his new community psychiatric nurse (CPN) began discussions with him to expand his life outside his mother's home. He mentioned that he used to run but didn't have the energy anymore and was too heavy. He confided in her concerns about his treatment and whether he would be able to stick to it in the long term.

> Box 8.1 Steps in exercise prescribing
>
> - An exercise prescription should consider the 'six As': assess, advise, agree, assist, arrange, and assess again.
> - Ask about your patient's physical activity regularly.
> - Categorize patients into frailty levels.
> - Consider a written prescription.
> - Get to know your local resources including sports/recreational clubs and fitness programmes, gyms, and certified fitness instructors.
> - Consider referrals to appropriate services, including within the multidisciplinary team (specialist physicians, physiotherapists, clinical exercise physiologists).
> - Follow-up to chart progress, set goals, solve problems, and identify and use social support.
>
> Adapted from *The BMJ*, 343, Khan, KM *et al*, Prescribing exercise in primary care: Ten practical steps on how to do it, Copyright (2011) with permission from BMJ Publishing Group Ltd.

She accompanied him to his next outpatient appointment where alternative treatment options were discussed. A change in medication was agreed. Even before this had begun he felt optimistic at the prospect. On his new medication he felt less hungry, had more energy, and began going for early morning walks. Within 2 months he was jogging for 15 minutes twice per week and had lost 4 kg. His paranoid symptoms were initially a little worse but diminished as he got to know the local area.

At his CPN's suggestion he entered a local fun run 2 months later. He began to run for longer in the evenings. He enjoyed the fun run and afterwards fell into conversation with an old friend. He was invited to join a group on their regular Sunday run. Within a year he had lost almost 15 kg and felt much fitter and more confident. Through one of his training partners he was offered a part-time job in local shop. He got on well with the staff and occasionally socialized with them after work.

Two years later he is still running regularly and competes in local road races. He enjoys the camaraderie of his work colleagues and the feeling that he is doing something useful.

Further reading

Almeida, O.P., Khan, K.M., Yeap, B.B., Golledge, J., and Flicker, L. (2014). 150 minutes of vigorous physical activity per week predicts survival and successful ageing: a population-based 11-year longitudinal study of 12 201 older Australian men. *Br J Sports Med* 48(3):220–5.

Anthony, W.A. (1993). Recovery from mental illness: the guiding vision of the mental health service system in the 1990s. *Psychosoc Rehabil J* 16:11–23.

Bailey, R. (2005). Evaluating the relationship between physical education, sport and social inclusion. *Educ Rev* 57(1):71–90.

Boardman, J., Currie, A., Killaspy, H., and Mezey, G. (2010). *Social Inclusion and Mental Health.* London: RCPsych Publications.

Caspersen, C.J., Powell, K.E., and Christenson, G.M. (1985). Physical activity, exercise, and physical fitness: definitions and distinctions for health-related research. *Public Health Rep* 100(2):126–31.

Donnelly, P. (1996). Approaches to social inequality in the sociology of sport. *Quest* 48:221–42.

Falkai, P., Malchow, B., Wobrock, T., Gruber, O., Schmitt, A., Honer, W.G., et al. (2013). The effect of aerobic exercise on cortical architecture in patients with chronic schizophrenia: a randomized controlled MRI study. *Eur Arch Psychiatry Clin Neurosci* 263(6):469–73.

Freiler, C. (2001). *What Needs to Change? Social Inclusion as a Focus of Wellbeing for Children, Families and Communities—A Draft Paper Concept.* Toronto, ON: Laidlaw Foundation.

Frew, E.J., Bhatti, M., Win, K., Sitch, A., Lyon, A., Pallan, M., et al. (2014). Cost-effectiveness of a community-based physical activity programme for adults (Be Active) in the UK: an economic analysis within a natural experiment. *Br J Sports Med* 48(3):207–12.

Ho, C.S.H., Zhang, M.W.B., Mak, A., and Ho, R.C.M. (2014). Metabolic syndrome in psychiatry: advances in understanding and management. *Adv Psychiatr Treat* 20:101–12.

Khan, K.M., Thompson, A.M., Blair, S.N., Sallis, J.F., Powell, K.E., Bull, F.C., et al. (2012). Sport and exercise as contributors to the health of nations. *Lancet* 380:59–64.

Khan, K.M., Weiler, R., and Blair, S.N. (2011). Prescribing exercise in primary care: ten practical steps on how to do it. *BMJ* 343:4141.

Mead, G.E., Morley, W., Campbell, P., Greig, C.A., McMurdo, M., and Lawlor, D.A. (2009). Exercise for depression. *Cochrane Database Syst Rev* 3:CD004366.

Penedo, F.J. and Dahn, J.R. (2005). Exercise and well-being: a review of mental and physical health benefits associated with physical activity. *Curr Opin Psychiatry* 18(2):189–93.

Websites

Mental Health Foundation: http://www.mentalhealth.org.uk

Royal College of Psychiatrists (Physical Activity and Mental Health): http://www.rcpsych.ac.uk/healthadvice/treatmentswellbeing/physicalactivity.aspx

UK Active: http://www.ukactive.com

Chapter 9

The sports arena

Kate Goodger and Sarah Broadhead

Key points

- The sports environment creates challenges for the work of the sports psychiatrist.
- The role of the sports psychiatrist can encompass working at several different levels: with individuals, teams, the sports environment, and sporting organizations.
- Sports psychiatry expertise can help athletes and coaches to get the most out of each phase of preparation and competition.
- Getting off to a good start within a sports team involves establishing boundaries and developing effective working relationships with coaches, athletes, and the support team.
- Time spent observing how the team works will pay dividends.
- Helping athletes with injuries will be a common occurrence and can be both proactive and reactive. Proactive help includes developing coping strategies before injury, whilst reactive interventions are directed at processing the event and planning for recovery and rehabilitation.

9.1 Introduction

The world of sport has its own cultural environment with accepted norms, values, beliefs, and behaviours. Moreover, many sports consider themselves unique in terms of culture and the physical, mental, technical, and tactical demands placed upon participants. An athlete presenting a mental health problem may experience similar symptoms to his/her non-athletic counterpart but these aspects of the environment of sport can affect the engagement of the athlete with a sports psychiatrist and, ultimately the outcome of this work.

Discussion of mental health problems remains difficult in many sports. Acknowledgement of mental health problems, or indeed working proactively to remain mentally healthy, is often considered to be a sign of weakness and simply less important than other aspects of training and competition. Sports psychology is a more established support service in the sports arena but continues to face challenges around the openness of athletes to working with these professionals. A feature that this discipline has exploited is that it can be seen to have a direct impact on performance. For the sports psychiatrist the prevention, treatment, and management of mental health is simply much harder to market at present.

A psychiatrist providing consultations to athletes with mental health problems will need to understand not only how these problems present but also the context in which they occur and the individuals they affect—the attributes of any good clinician. A psychiatrist seeking a role as an integral member of the support team of sports medical and sports science practitioners who work in high-performance sport may find that not only are these opportunities relatively rare but also that they necessitate a different way of working and a detailed understanding of the sports arena. This chapter aims to provide some practical guidance on how to begin working with athletes and sports teams, the possible scope of the work clinicians can undertake, and the potential to extend this beyond the traditional mental health remit.

9.2 Getting off to a good start

There are a few important practical considerations for sports psychiatrists that can improve their chances of engaging athletes and establishing themselves as a valued support service within a sports team or organization.

9.2.1 Boundaries and establishing your role

It is helpful to develop an answer to the commonly asked question 'What is it you do then?'. Although sports psychiatry is focused on mental health issues and problems, it is not necessarily exclusive to this. For example, a psychiatrist can improve athletic performance by helping athletes to develop emotional skills. It is valuable to be able to quote everyday examples of the added value of sports psychiatry approaches like this. It is useful to be able to do this without using jargon so that sports psychiatry methods are seen as accessible and uncomplicated. Examples include:

• developing confidence
• managing relationships
• communicating effectively
• managing rest and recovery
• coping with adversity
• consistency in training
• optimizing concentration and attention.

From the outset it is important to establish who the client is and what is expected in supporting their needs. Goal posts can quickly shift in sport and it is important to know:

• where the role starts and finishes
• what is the remit and key responsibilities associated with the role?
• what are the key objectives?
• how will these be measured?

It's not unusual for a clinician to be asked to roll their sleeves up and carry the water bottles or hold the video camera for a coach during a training session. This also helps to build rapport and approachability, and gets people used to a sports psychiatrist being around.

9.2.2 **Confidentiality**

Confidentiality can make coaches and other members of an athlete's support team uncomfortable. There may be a mystique around the role of the sports psychiatrist (and perhaps others in the support team too) where it is perceived that practitioners are being deliberately and unhelpfully secretive. A coach may complain that she/he 'simply doesn't know what these people do with my athletes'.

As with any other patient, the athlete and sports psychiatrist have a confidential clinician–patient relationship where the normal rules of patient confidentiality apply. However, there is an added complication in that the sports psychiatrist may be an employee of the sports organization and subject to the terms agreed at the commencement of employment. A practitioner can have two masters: firstly, the athlete/patient and secondly, the team or organization and its management. In high-performance or professional sports there may be protocols or contracts where the athlete signs a disclosure agreement. It is essential to understand any existing procedures for managing confidentiality. If there are none then permission must obtained from the athlete/patient before any disclosures and a process agreed on how information will be shared beyond the doctor–patient relationship if this is required. This is particularly pertinent in situations when a referral is made by a third party (e.g. a coach referring an athlete, or a team manager referring a coach) and when there is an expectation of some element of feedback to the referrer.

Perhaps the most important aspect of doctor–patient confidentiality is to ensure that it is managed effectively day to day and does not become a bone of contention for support staff. This includes being open about confidentiality, highlighting that it is fundamental to the practice of medicine. It is not designed to deliberately conceal but rather to afford privacy. If the clinician is also proactive in encouraging athletes to share what is appropriate and involves relevant support staff as needed, with the permission of the athlete, confidentiality can quickly become an accepted and respected mode of operation.

Case study 1

A 20-year-old swimmer has a mental health issue which the sports psychiatrist is helping him to manage. The coach has asked the sports psychiatrist to feed into a selection meeting with any information that could impact on the selection decision for this athlete to travel to an 8-week training camp overseas.

The sports psychiatrist asked the swimmer what he was willing to share with the coach and other support staff. The swimmer was happy to be open about issues he was dealing with in his private life, as he had a good relationship with the team around him and felt it would be helpful for them to know. The swimmer did not want to go into details but was happy for them to know it was a sensitive time.

The sports psychiatrist and swimmer had a meeting with the sport team to help them understand that they were doing ongoing work on personal issues as well as performance-related work. The sports psychiatrist and swimmer believed that the swimmer could function well on the training camp if given access to support from the psychiatrist whilst away.

9.2.3 **Observing**

Working in the sports arena can evoke a response in the sports psychiatrist to be 'active' and 'get involved' but there is valuable time spent in observing everyday behaviours around the training and competition environment. It is critically important to get to know the environment, the culture, what the climate is like, who does what, when, and how, and so on. In the practice or training environment, coaches may ask for feedback on sessions and this can provide a useful point of entry to working with them. It is also a chance to establish a baseline comparison of how individuals operate in their everyday environment and compare this with their performance under the pressure of competition. It is not unusual for coaches to describe athletes who are 'great trainers but can't compete on the day' or to report frustrations with athletes 'who don't put the work in during training but are able to pull it out of the bag on the day'.

9.3 **Managing relationships**

A critical skill of the sports psychiatrist is to build and maintain relationships. Initially at least this may be done opportunistically and during brief contacts. Conversations can happen in the dinner queue or on the team bus. These can sometimes be significant interactions that lay the foundations for future productive working relationships. Within the athlete's 'sports family' there will be a number of significant people and it is worthwhile to know who they are and what their role is.

9.3.1 **Working with coaches**

Arguably the most important relationship in an athlete's sports career is with their coach. Most likely this is the person they will spend most time with, who has the greatest influence, and who will have the biggest impact on performance. Often the coach is the 'gate-keeper' to working with an athlete and failing to have an effective working relationship with a coach can have a significant detrimental effect on any work done with an athlete. Equally, a respected coach can be one of the best advocates for the work of a sports psychiatrist.

Coaches show great variability in their approach and it is important to take time to get to know a coach, their way of working, and how they want you to work. A coach may feel threatened or become territorial towards a sports psychiatrist if they believe they are better placed to work mentally with an athlete. This may indeed be the case and some coaches offer very high levels of personal and emotional support and are skilled in mentally preparing athletes for competition. However, there are also dysfunctional coach–athlete relationships where the coach can contribute to an athlete's anxieties, and complications such as when a coach and athlete enter into a romantic relationship.

Establishing roles with coaches

It is important for the sports psychiatrist to be clear about their own role and to establish the ground rules of working with a coach and athlete. This can be done by:

• looking at ways of working with the coach and their athlete together
• agreeing key objectives for the work that will be undertaken
• establishing how progress will be measured
• agreeing how communication and updates will be provided

- providing training to coaches (professional development) to help them to support their athlete's needs
- supporting coaches in managing any occupational stresses associated with their role.

9.3.2 **Sports science and sports medicine teams**

It is increasingly common in high-performance sports for there to be a multidisciplinary team of practitioners who provide support services to athletes. Broadly these practitioners fit into two groups:

1. Sport science practitioners including professionals in the fields of:

   - strength and conditioning
   - biomechanics and performance analysis
   - performance nutrition
   - sports psychology
   - performance lifestyle.

2. Sports medicine practitioners who may include:

   - chief medical officer or team doctor
   - physiotherapist
   - clinical psychologist.

Sports psychiatrist

It is important that the role of the sports psychiatrist is clear and explicit. This will avoid blurring of boundaries and duplication, or creating gaps because of an assumption that someone else was doing it. This is especially important in a team where a sports psychiatrist is employed alongside a sports or clinical psychologist, although it would be unusual if a sport were to employ all three practitioners. The sports psychiatrist would expect to deal with most psychiatric conditions but there can be confusion if the psychiatrist is also providing either therapeutic support (that could be provided by a clinical psychologist), or performance-enhancement approaches (that may be within the scope of a sports psychologist).

In a sport where there is no 'in-house' sports psychiatrist then support for the assessment and treatment of most psychiatric disorders would be by a referral from the medical team to an appropriate specialist. If there are other practitioners involved it is important to understand how they want to operate and what the sport requires.

Clinical psychologist

Clinical psychologists aim to improve the psychological well-being of their clients. They use psychological methods, research, and a variety of treatments to help their clients make positive changes to their lives. The background and training of a clinical psychologist is focused on areas such as:

- depression and anxiety
- adjustment to physical illness

- neurological disorders
- addictive behaviours
- challenging behaviours
- eating disorders
- personal and family relationship problems
- learning disabilities.

Sports psychologist

Practitioners may have trained under the supervision of the British Psychological Society or the British Association of Sport and Exercise Science to become, respectively, either chartered or certified sports psychologists. They may focus on how sport and exercise participation affects health and well-being. However, in competitive sport a key role is to support performance enhancement through mental or psychological skills. Examples of this type of work include:

- communication
- confidence
- goal setting
- imagery
- relaxation
- performance routines
- self-talk
- planning
- attentional control.

Avoiding the sweetie shop effect

Some athletes feel at a disadvantage if they do not have access to all of the same personnel and facilities as others. Some behave like 'a kid in a sweetie shop', accessing too many services to gauge the impact of each and others may become reliant on services.

A sports psychiatrist will need to establish the skills, roles, and responsibilities of other members of the support team. This applies to all members of the team not just the sports science and sports medicine practitioners. This helps in several ways:

- To execute professional courtesies around roles and sharing of information
- To understand the landscape for the athlete
- To avoid over- or under-providing for athletes.

Case study 2

A sports psychologist has been working in a sport for 8 years and become an established member of the support staff. A sports psychiatrist has recently been recruited to support the mental health needs of athletes and staff. The sports psychologist is concerned that this will mean an encroachment on their territory and they are reluctant to engage with the sports psychiatrist.

The two arrange to meet to discuss the outcomes they and the team want for the athletes. They both share a desire for the athletes to be performing at their best and to be in optimum physical and mental health. They discuss their respective areas of expertise and the sports psychiatrist acknowledges the wide-ranging knowledge of the athletes and team that the sports psychologist has built up over the 8-year period.

They later discuss several cases and by focusing on the needs of the athlete are able to allocate areas for each to concentrate on. In some cases, involvement of the sports psychiatrist will not be needed and in others the sports psychologist will not have an active role. By working in this way they recognize the benefits of communication and agree to meet for regular discussions.

9.3.3 **Athlete support network**

The support network around athletes is often critical to success. This was recognized at the London 2012 Olympics by a commercially sponsored 'Friends and Family' initiative for Team GB athletes. This provided resources and services for the athlete's extended support network to help in their preparations for the Games.

When working with an athlete it is valuable to develop a clear idea of the make-up of their support network at an early stage. Who do they go to for help and advice? Who do they spend time with inside and outside their sport? Which are the most significant relationships to them? How are family and friends involved in their sport?

The sports psychiatrist may be asked to work with members of an athlete's support network to assist an athlete with a particular problem or circumstance. If work is required within an athlete's support network, it is once again advisable to establish boundaries and expectations for this work.

It is more common for the psychiatrist to be working with the athlete as an individual and supporting them in managing situations and relationships in their life. An athlete's beliefs about themselves, their self-image, self-esteem, and self-worth are often linked to significant relationships and past episodes. In this respect they are no different to non-athletes. An important area of work therefore may be to help athletes deal with past and current problems and their potential impact on current behaviours, beliefs, and emotions.

Case study 3

A 28-year-old male rower has begun working with a sports psychiatrist after acknowledging an ongoing battle for many years with low self-esteem, anxiety, and low mood. On asking him why he does his sport he answers that it has always been to prove a point to his father that he was much more able than his father had given him credit for.

The sports psychiatrist asked the rower how he wanted to be and what he wanted to base his self-esteem on. After discussions and reflection the rower said he would like to base his self-esteem on his own life values. These values were doing your best and being proud of the effort you put in, regardless of outcome. He recognized these were different values to his father's, and that he couldn't change those. The rower decided he would work on reinforcing his own values and not taking his father's comments personally. By accepting that it is normal to seek approval from parents, but not always helpful, this helped deal with the situation. They discussed whether the rower wanted to involve his father in any sessions but concluded this was not something he wanted to do at this point.

9.4 **Working with teams**

Working with a team of athletes presents different rewards and challenges to those of working with individual athletes. At an early stage it is important to understand the features of the team. These include the more formalized elements such as team structure, operating procedures for training and competition, and individual roles and responsibilities within these frameworks. Alongside this it is necessary to become aware of the less formalized elements that constitute the 'team dynamic'. These include the nature of individual communications and interactions, the prevailing mood or 'feeling' within the team, and the accepted behaviours and underlying values. The 'team culture' includes aspects of the more structured components, of 'how things are done around here', and of the teams' and team members' underpinning beliefs and values. Understanding all of this is fundamental to working with the team. Opportunities for exploring this can happen through observing:

- team meetings
- team talks
- pre-competition processes
- the organization of training
- performance debriefs
- feedback processes from both players and coaches around performance.

Understanding a team's approach and how it operates collectively and across individual members, helps to identify sources of potential dysfunction in a team's dynamic. It also affords the opportunity to enhance mental well-being and performance by establishing a functional and cohesive dynamic.

In addition to spending time getting to know the team and the different constituent personalities it is also helpful to assess and identify key roles within the team. Leadership and in particular its level of visibility, impact, and effectiveness is an important role for a practitioner to explore and assess. Other key roles within a team are the 'cultural architects'. This term was introduced to the England national football team in the early 2000s by a Norwegian sports psychologist, Professor Willi Railo. The architects are those team members able to build a functional and strong team dynamic from within. They typically possess leadership attributes, are role models or senior/experienced team members, and have impact and influence over their peers. Being able to establish a good relationship with the cultural architects significantly enhances the engagement of the whole team whilst failing to do so will compromise this task.

Case study 4

The head coach of a rugby team wants to work with a sports psychiatrist to create a leadership culture within his squad. He is frustrated that players do not take on leadership responsibilities. For example, when pressure mounts on the pitch the team do not communicate effectively and go within themselves.

Assessment: the sports psychiatrist gathered information to assess the team culture. The head coach was interviewed to establish what culture he wanted and why. All squad members and staff were also interviewed. Understanding these collective views resulted in a formulation of the problem and a description of the challenges.

Intervention: the sports psychiatrist wanted the whole team to engage with the need for a different culture. A series of facilitated group sessions were used to explore what the new culture and its benefits could be. Barriers to this were also discussed, openly highlighting the importance of a safe discussion environment to encourage honesty. The sports psychiatrist carefully planned the sessions, taking into account the dynamics of the team and using the cultural architects to help the sessions run more smoothly. A set of behaviours was agreed that would be regularly reviewed and reinforced by all. The sports psychiatrist also worked one-to-one with the head coach to help manage his frustration and to develop a more proactive approach that he could use to encourage the desired behaviours within the squad.

Outcome: the head coach had a clearer view of the outcome he wanted and the challenges to achieving this. After the one-to-one sessions he was able to manage frustrations more effectively and support the team to implement the behaviours that were agreed. Communication levels within the team were observed to be better before, during, and after games.

9.5 **Injury**

Injury is a fact of life in sport but the impact and consequences of an injury mean that these are highly significant events for athletes. Injury leads to non-participation with implications not just for the athlete themselves but also potential consequences (or perceived consequences) to those around them including coaches, teammates, team managers, sponsors, family, and friends. Indeed, working with injured athletes is uniquely challenging because of the potential impact of what in other circumstances might be a relatively trivial ailment of limited significance.

The benefits for an athlete in working psychologically on injury-related issues are broad and encompass:

- injury vulnerability.
- rehabilitation and recovery.
- return to sport.
- transition out of sport if the injury is career ending.

The role of the sports psychiatrist can therefore be proactive around injury prevention and injury prehab (building strength in areas of injury vulnerability), as well as reactive once an injury has occurred.

9.5.1 **Vulnerability to injury**

Psychological and psychosocial factors linked to injury susceptibility and vulnerability include:

- stressors (major life events, daily hassles, and previous injury history)
- personality (perfectionism, an external locus of control, and mood states such as anxiety)
- coping resources (having poor coping skills and a weak support network).

Preventative interventions reduce susceptibility by developing mental skills such as relaxation, stress management, goal setting, imagery, and attentional control, whilst cognitive behavioural techniques can enhance self-esteem, confidence, and improve the athlete's stress response.

9.5.2 **Rehabilitation and recovery**

Athlete responses to injury can be both complex and varied. Two broad types of responses have been described:

1. *Intrapersonal psychological responses comprising:*

   * cognitions—for example, attributions for injury occurrence, appraisal of the injury, and its implications
   * emotions—these span immediate responses to the injury as well as responses to both progress and setbacks during the rehabilitation process and positive and negatives emotions associated with returning to sport
   * behaviours—including those around coping skills and adherence to the rehabilitation programme.

2. *Interpersonal interactions and the response of others.* These relevant and important interactions are usually focused within the patient–practitioner relationship but may also extend to other relationships including with the coach and teammates:

   * Helping athletes to feel there is a support process in place is hugely beneficial.
   * Athletes often want 'black and white' answers which medical teams are unable to provide. Support with managing this uncertainty is key. The sports psychiatrist can work alongside the medical team to ensure the athlete fully understands the injury and healing process.
   * Anxiety about the impact of missed training sessions is also common and understandable. The sports psychiatrist can assist athletes to find helpful coping strategies.
   * Injured athletes can feel excluded from their sport due to the enforced change in their routine. They may experience social isolation, for example, if they are attending physiotherapy sessions by themselves. Large gaps in their schedule can result in significant boredom that needs to be managed. Consideration needs to be given on how to help athletes maintain their relationship with their sport and teammates and to manage their time.

9.5.3 **Return to sport**

Physical healing does not necessarily coincide completely with an athlete's psychological readiness to return to sport. The transition back into sport can be complicated by anxieties around whether pre-injury performance levels can be met, the threat of re-injury, meeting expectations of self and others, loss of identity, feeling disconnected from the sport and the team, and coercion to return prematurely.

For some athletes being injured can evoke a response not unlike a grief reaction. There is a perception of a significant loss whether this is the ability to do something they love or the impact on achieving sporting goals. Athletes often exhibit:

* denial—'It's not as bad as the medical team say it is'
* anger—'It's not fair that I am injured, I always get injured, I will miss selection'
* bargaining—negotiating with coaches or medical team about return to training or competition
* depression—'It's hopeless; I'll never be able to get back to fitness'

- acceptance—with commitment to a helpful plan.

Positive engagement will support an athlete through this process and enhance rehabilitation and eventual return to sport (or transition out of sport if the injury is career ending).

9.6 **Training**

The daily training environment provides mental challenges for athletes. Therefore sports psychiatrists have a role in addressing these challenges with athletes and coaches and maximizing training benefits. Sports psychiatrists can help athletes and coaches to set objectives for each session and then carry out an effective debrief to review these objectives and support the learning process.

It is helpful to understand the psychological approach and mindset that will ensure optimum returns from any training session. In addition, it can be useful to think through the disadvantages and pitfalls of failing to achieve the desired mindset. For example, a runner may wish to complete a set of repetition runs with the objective of giving a maximal effort in each run. A common pitfall is to hold back on the first few repetitions to conserve energy for the later runs. The sports psychiatrist can use an understanding of the mind to make the athlete aware of what is happening and devising strategies to avoid this. Other training issues that may need to be addressed are lack of motivation, not having clear objectives for each session, dwelling on mistakes and getting frustrated, unhelpful rivalry with teammates, and disagreements and arguments with the coach.

9.7 **Competing**

It is helpful to think of three phases of competition. These are the pre- and post-competition phases and the competition itself.

9.7.1 **Pre competition**

Preparation before an event is critical to success in the environment of competition. This is not simply training and rehearsal to achieve physical and technical readiness but also preparation of the mind. Preparatory work helps athletes develop effective competition plans and to practise and test the skills and strategies for use in important events.

Work in this area can include:

- determining goals for the event (often months or years ahead)
- contingency planning ('What if . . . ?')
- establishing routines for use in competition (e.g. pre-performance routines)
- expectation management
- distraction management
- mental warm-up and cool-down
- post-performance evaluation after preparatory events leading up to the major competition
- staying healthy (e.g. hygiene around the venue, dining facilities, sleep, rest, and recovery)
- familiarization (e.g. the competition venue, the event schedule, and regulations for accreditation and doping control).

9.7.2 **During competition**

It is important to fully understand the demands of the competition environment and agree the times when the sports psychiatrist will support the athlete and coach at the event itself and what methods will be used. It is useful to be aware that the behaviours and thought processes of athlete, coach, and support team member can change and become unpredictable in the competition environment. In response to this, pre-agreed plans and methods may need to be altered at short notice. A team may work and live in close proximity to each other for extended periods and this can strain otherwise good relationships. The sports psychiatrist will need to be alert to this and ready to intervene and exert a calming influence when necessary.

9.7.3 **Post competition—debriefing**

The sports psychiatrist can be useful in coordinating or facilitating the debrief process for the athlete/coach or team after an important event. Often the initial response is an emotional one (either positive or negative depending on the result) rather than objectively based. The expression of emotion is important so a later and more objective review might also need to take place. An athlete may go through a process not unlike a grief reaction after a disappointing performance or perceived underachievement. The sports psychiatrist role can help achieve a balanced and realistic perspective and then refocus on learning lessons to incorporate into longer-term plans (see Box 9.1).

Paradoxically, athletes can also experience emotional lows even after a victory. Some may report feeling pressure to repeat that performance or worry they have 'peaked too soon' before a major event. If they are successful at an event they have been working towards for a long time they can report loss of focus and motivation to carry on training afterwards.

9.8 **Not just mental health**

Although supporting the mental health of an athlete is the central role of the sports psychiatrist the work need not be limited to this area. Optimizing how athletes function has scope extending beyond the field of play and the clinician can make a significant impact in shaping the nature of the environment that surrounds an athlete.

Among the most successful example of this approach has been the work of Steve Peters with British Cycling and Team Sky (the professional road cycling team) alongside Dave Brailsford the performance director of both teams. Brailsford has described the task 'to create a culture of support for the riders. To *really* support them, so that they can be the best that they can be'. The employment of a psychiatrist was to help create an approach and system that emphasized the rider as whole person and looked beyond the traditional focus on training and performance alone.

The role of the sports psychiatrist working in this way can be understood by considering a framework where she/he has input at several different levels. These include:

- the individual
- the team
- the environment
- the organization.

Box 9.1 An example of a structured event debrief when working with an athlete and coach

Purpose
To support continuous improvement by reviewing the mental components of racing.

Mindset and race plan
Fill in the table below with red/amber/green (RAG) ratings for each component and for each stage of the race and reflecting your effort level and delivery (Del) of performance. You can watch the video analysis to remind yourself of each part of the race.

	1st round heat		2nd round heat		Semi-final		Final	
	Effort	Del	Effort	Del	Effort	Del	Effort	Del
Mindset on the start line	G	G						
Clear race plan	G	G						
Full commitment to race plan	G	G						
Delivery of race plan	G	G						
No. of key refocus points	1							
Main reasons for key refocusing	Unhelpful thoughts on outcome		1.		1.		1.	
Speed of refocusing	A							

Athletes notes: *I was clear on my race plan and cue points. It went well until I made a mistake and thought how this would affect the time. I refocused on the next cue point, reminding myself this would give me the best chance, but was a little slow to refocus.*
Key: RAG = Red, Amber, Green.
Red = off track or deteriorating trend.
Amber = making progress but inconsistent or a concern has emerged which needs addressing.
Green = on track and making expected or better progress.

9.8.1 **The individual**

When working with individual athletes the focus is on developing skills to manage emotions. Initially this may be primarily to aid performance but athletes have a life beyond sport that can affect their well-being and ability to focus in training and competition. The sports psychiatrist's role can extend into these areas to develop coping strategies for a life outside of sport. The athlete can be helped to develop mental skills in areas such as:

• managing pressure
• managing expectations

- dealing with success and failure
- dealing with setbacks
- commitment
- confidence.

The psychiatrist may also work individually with other members of the support team. Additional areas that can be addressed when working with staff members include:

- dealing with relationship difficulties
- personal and professional crisis
- managing requirements of their role.

9.8.2 **The team**

Working with a team may mean working with a competitive team or perhaps a training squad or the staff and support team around an athlete. Specific difficulties that may arise from being part of a team include selection issues, competition for roles, contracts, playing time, and leadership and management decision-making (e.g. who has accreditations at sporting events, and who is hired and fired from the team). All of these difficulties can result in emotional reactions from athletes and staff, which the sports psychiatrist can play a role in helping to prevent and manage.

Effective communication and managing relationships are important areas to consider. Conflict within staff teams can be a major distraction during training and competition. Time spent establishing systems to manage conflict ahead of key competitions may prove invaluable later. This can include ensuring there is clarity and acceptance around roles and responsibilities with an explicit chain of command, well-rehearsed operating procedures, contingency/crisis management plans, and consistent, clear communication.

9.8.3 **The environment**

The environmental tier is focused on creating the optimal performance climate around an athlete in training and competition. The environment around an athlete includes the physical environment (e.g. training base), personnel (members of the support team and their roles), and having a clear planning and review process. The environment is influenced by factors including:

- clarity of leadership
- effective communication systems
- effective goal setting and planning
- clear and well-communicated expectations
- clear and well-understood roles, responsibilities, and operating processes.

9.8.4 **The organization**

Most organizations have a mission (a reason for existing) and associated values and beliefs. Sports teams and organizations are just the same as any other business in many ways. The leader of the organization and the culture they create will have a massive impact on the environment, the team, and the individuals that sit within it. Culture is 'how we do things around here' and the behaviours that are acceptable and encouraged.

The sports psychiatrist can have an influence and input at the organizational level. If a stable and helpful culture is created then this can greatly help individuals to thrive and develop. For example, sports psychiatrists can help create a culture that is always looking for ways to improve, or a culture that encourages open and honest discussion of thoughts and feelings.

9.9 **Key questions**

These questions will help the sports psychiatrist to develop their approach to working with athletes and coaches.

From the psychiatrist:

- How can the impact of my work be measured?
- What will I actually be doing with athletes?
- How will I manage confidentiality?
- How is what I do different to working with a sports psychologist?

From others:

- What has mental health got to do with sport, you are either tough enough or you're not?
- How can you help me as a coach get more out of my athletes?
- Isn't there a danger that you're going to create dependency in your athletes?
- What does a typical session look like for an athlete and how long do you need?
- How does sitting and talking about stuff in an office transfer to the sports arena?
- Plenty of athletes succeed without all this mental stuff, do athletes really need it?
- Tell me what you can do for my team in the time it takes me to drink this coffee?

Further reading

Brukner, P. and Khan, K. (Eds.) (2007). *Clinical Sports Medicine* (3rd ed.). Australia: McGraw-Hill.

Heil, J. and Podlog, L. (2012). Injury and performance. In Murphy. S.M. (Ed.), The *Oxford Handbook of Sport and Exercise Psychology* (pp. 593–617). New York: Oxford University Press.

Moore, R. (2008). *Heroes, Villains and Velodromes: Chris Hoy and Britain's Track Cycling Revolution.* London: Harper Sport.

Chapter 10

Psychotropic drug prescribing

Allan Johnston and R. Hamish McAllister-Williams

Key points

- Doctors and other medical staff have an overriding need to treat those who are ill. Thoughtful prescribing on an individual basis can often achieve this without compromising athletic performance.
- Follow good prescribing practices as in any other clinical area.
- There are special considerations when prescribing psychotropic drugs to those who are exercising intensively and repeatedly.
- There is little evidence to guide specific drug choices for athletes. Consider the drug's pharmacology, pharmacokinetics, and side effect profile.
- Be aware of the regulations regarding drug use in any sport and the need for Therapeutic Use Exemptions.

10.1 Introduction

Good psychotropic drug prescribing in elite sport shares much with good prescribing practice in all other fields of healthcare. Good prescribing is based on a review of the relevant evidence base, a consideration of the situation of the individual patient, and clinical experience. All this occurs in a framework of appropriate clinical governance. It relies on sound clinical skills, care, compassion, and the prescriber–patient relationship. The needs of the individual patient must be paramount in this relationship. Issues of aftercare and monitoring for adverse effects should be well planned and thorough. Despite the rapid pace of modern drug development we should pay heed to longstanding counsel: *primum non nocere*—first do no harm.

There may be additional factors to consider in prescribing for elite athletes:

- The particular sport and its demands
- The level of performance required
- Physiological and biochemical characteristics, including past medical history
- The avoidance of any pharmacokinetic or pharmacodynamic effects that may impede performance. Athletes suffering from mental health problems invariably have reservations about taking medication with unknown effects on safety and performance.

This chapter seeks to explore these issues, using all available evidence in the field. The aim is to illustrate that psychotropic drug prescribing in sports is a matter of general good clinical practice allied to additional considerations about the context in which prescribing will occur. Whilst there is a need to avoid side effects that may impact elite performance there is an overriding need to provide adequate treatment for any mental health problem.

10.2 **Factors to consider when choosing the right drug for the individual**

The term 'sport' covers a wide range of meanings and activities. Limiting ourselves to the 'games or activities for pleasure', there is in the region of 8000 sports and sporting games across the world. They are as diverse as rugby league, rhythmic gymnastics, cross-country skiing, and beach volleyball. Each sport presents a variety of challenges in terms of the physical demands, environment, timing, duration, and mental strengths required. Even within the same team, athletes may face very different demands: from the opening batsman to the fast bowler in a cricket team, and from the oarsman to the coxswain in a rowing crew. Sports are played by individuals of differing age, size, gender, ethnicity, religion, health, and disability. Therefore, there is a complex range of pharmacokinetic and pharmacodynamic considerations with every individual and with every prescription.

10.2.1 **Pharmacokinetics**

Pharmacokinetics describe how the body processes a specific drug. This includes the absorption, physical distribution, metabolism, and excretion of that substance. Differences between individual athletes can be of great importance.

Absorption

Factors affecting the rate of drug absorption include the formulation of the drug and the physical state of the athlete, for example, the area of absorptive surface, the pH of gastric fluid, the degree of gastrointestinal motility, and vascularity (during intense exercise blood is preferentially shunted away from the gut towards large muscle groups). Conditions such as coeliac or Crohn's disease can also have important effects on the rate of gastrointestinal absorption.

With an oral drug, the timing of administration is important and must achieve not only the desired effect but also avoid adverse or unwanted effects. In many sports, caffeinated products such as energy drinks or gels are widely used to enhance performance. A mistimed dose may leave the athlete with post-match restlessness, even insomnia, and without any objective benefit to performance. As an example, a high-profile FIFA World Cup qualifying match was postponed minutes before kick-off as a result of torrential rain. The football match was rescheduled the following day but the visiting team underperformed and did not achieve the expected result. It was reported that the players had used caffeine tablets before the postponed match, had then required sleeping tablets that evening, and then more caffeine tablets the following day. As with most things in sport, timing is everything.

Distribution

All drugs distribute between the lipid, protein, and water components of the body. Most psychotropic drugs are lipid-soluble (which allows them to penetrate the blood–brain barrier and reach their site of action) and their volume of distribution is affected by relative adiposity or leanness. Many athletes are lean and there is theoretically a smaller volume of distribution for lipid-soluble psychotropic drugs in these individuals. When the volume of distribution of a drug is reduced, corresponding dose reductions may need to be considered. However, the therapeutic window (i.e. the difference between the minimum effective concentration and level above which side effects predominate) is relatively wide for most psychotropics, especially antidepressants, and therefore it is sensible to start with standard doses but monitor for side effects. Few psychotropic drugs are water-soluble and so the state of an athlete's hydration (e.g. dehydration as an endurance event progresses or in a boxer struggling to make weight) is a less common consideration. Lithium prescribing is considered in more detail in Section 10.3.2.

Metabolism

Drug metabolism occurs largely in the liver to produce water-soluble metabolites that allow excretion in urine or bile. Hepatic metabolism can be profoundly affected by any substance that the athlete is already using. A full history should be taken from the athlete of all medications including over-the-counter medications. Many drugs induce the hepatic enzymes that produce soluble metabolites and this will accelerate the metabolism and excretion of other drugs. Conversely, drugs that inhibit hepatic enzymes will slow the metabolism and excretion of co-administered drugs. Advice from national formularies such as the British National Formulary should be sought with regard to drug interactions. Two helpful mnemonics are 'PCGRABS' for enzyme inducers and 'SHOPTHEM' for enzyme inhibitors (see Table 10.1).

Excretion

Psychotropic drugs are excreted largely by the kidneys in a process involving glomerular filtration, active secretion, and passive tubular reabsorption. The half-life of a drug (the time taken for half of the remaining drug concentration to be eliminated) is affected by a range of physiological, pathological, and environmental factors. A sufficient degree of hydration is important not only for optimal athletic performance but also for adequate drug excretion. Hydration is a particularly important issue for drugs that are not metabolized and exist free in body water such as lithium (see Section 10.3.2). An athlete's hydration needs will relate to the duration and intensity of performance in addition to the playing environment. For example, the environmental challenges of the 2018 FIFA World Cup in Russia will be quite different to those in the following competition scheduled for summer 2022 in Qatar. Senior officials have already raised concerns about the extreme heat in that Gulf state.

10.2.2 **Pharmacodynamics**

The pharmacodynamics of a drug describe the effect of the drug on the body. This includes the desirable biochemical and physiological effects of a drug that largely occur through effects on receptors or second messenger systems. Clearly all athletes desire a beneficial effect and symptomatic improvement; partly as a result of the inconvenience of scheduling medication into a busy training timetable and partly as a counterbalance to any side effects experienced. This is simply a cost/benefit calculation. Minimizing any undesirable effects or adverse reactions of drug treatment is critical to a high-performing athlete who does not want treatment to compromise performance.

Table 10.1 Drug effects on hepatic enzymes	
Hepatic enzyme inducers	
Drug/class	Example
P Phenytoin	
C Carbamazepine	
G Griseofulvin	
R Rifampicin	
A Alcohol	
B Barbituates	Phenobarbital
S Smoking	Nicotine
Hepatic enzyme inhibitors	
Drug/class	Example
S SSRIs	Sertraline
H Haloperidol	
O Other antibiotics	Trimethoprim
P Phenothiazine antipsychotics	Chlorpromazine
T Tricyclic antidepressants	Amitriptyline
H Histamine H$_2$ antagonists	Ranitidine
E Erythromycin	
M Monoamine-oxidase inhibitor antidepressants	Moclobemide

Adverse drug reactions can be categorized as the following:

• Intolerance—expected or recognized side effects that may be dose related
• Idiosyncratic—unexpected or unrecognized side effects inconsistent with the known pharmacology of the drug
• Allergic—side effects modulated by the immune system as a result of predisposition
• Drug interaction—side effects as a result of one drug's effect on another. This can be direct (a pharmacodynamic drug interaction) or indirect via an effect on the body (a pharmacokinetic drug interaction).

Good clinical practice requires assessment of the risks and benefits of any treatment and a discussion with the athlete. In order to obtain informed consent to proceed, sufficient information must be provided to allow the athlete to understand and weigh up the pros and cons of any proposed treatment. As a minimum, all common and potentially serious side effects should be discussed. There may be guidelines available to support this choice, for example, the UK's National Institute of Health and Care Excellence (NICE) guidance available at http://www.nice.org.uk.

Particular side effects of psychotropic medications to consider in an athlete include the following:

- Cognitive—sedation, drowsiness, or impaired concentration
- Motor—tremor, rigidity, akathisia, or bradykinesia
- Weight—gain or loss relating to changes in appetite
- Visual—blurred vision or dizziness
- Psychological—anxiety or agitation
- Sleep—insomnia, abnormal dreams, or morning sedation (a 'hangover' effect)
- Cardiac—postural hypotension, hypertension, tachycardia, palpitations, arrhythmias, or electrocardiogram (ECG) changes such as QTc prolongation—a marker for the risk of ventricular tachyarrhythmias.

10.3 **Evidence base and choice of psychotropic drug**

While there is a substantial evidence base supporting, for example, the use of antidepressants to treat depression or anxiety disorders and antipsychotics in the treatment of psychosis or mania, there is a paucity of research specifically looking at the use of psychotropic drugs in athletes. What data there is was reviewed by Reardon and Factor in 2010. Existing evidence has usually been obtained in small, unreplicated studies and by examining acute effects of single doses of medication. As psychotropic medication is usually prescribed for months or longer this makes translating the evidence base even more a matter of clinical judgement.

10.3.1 **Antidepressants**

Selective serotonin reuptake inhibitors (SSRIs) are the first-line treatments for depression and anxiety disorders when severity warrants medication. This is probably the case for athletes as well and fluoxetine seems to be the antidepressant most commonly prescribed by psychiatrists for sportspeople. There is little data on the effect of SSRIs on performance. There have been suggestions that SSRIs may attenuate the endorphin release that occurs during and just after exercise and conflicting reports on their effect on time to exhaustion (increases and decreases have both been observed). Limited evidence suggests that paroxetine might increase core body temperature, creating a risk of problematic overheating in endurance events in hot conditions. All of these findings have been made following at most two doses of medication and there is no data on the repeated dosing that would be expected in clinical practice. Recent evidence from a large meta-analysis of 117 studies and 26 000 participants demonstrated that sertraline is marginally more effective than other antidepressants, and is well tolerated. It also does not cause QTc prolongation. This makes it a logical first-choice SSRI for many athletes (see Table 10.2).

There is even less data regarding the use of other classes of antidepressants in athletes. There are no randomized trials of tricyclic antidepressants and sedating effects mean they are not ideal choices. Pro-cardiac arrhythmic effects are also theoretical reasons for caution. It is reported that reboxetine may decrease athletic performance but the observations were made after a single dose not representative of usual clinical practice. Bupropion is licensed as an antidepressant in some countries but not in Europe. Studies of single doses in athletic populations show mixed findings with one suggesting that it might improve aerobic performance in hot conditions. This, along with other concerns regarding its stimulant effects, means that it is under review as a potentially prohibited substance.

For all other antidepressants there is no meaningful data on effects and safety in athletes. From a theoretical standpoint, agomelatine should be considered a suitable antidepressant (see Table 10.2). It is taken at night and has a half-life of around 90 minutes meaning there are negligible levels in the body during waking hours and consequently few side effects. However, it causes hepatic dysfunction and liver function tests are required before treatment and to monitor for dysfunction with repeat tests at 3, 6, 12, and 24 weeks.

10.3.2 **Antipsychotics and mood stabilizers**

Managing bipolar disorder in athletes is a major challenge. In many situations, second-generation antipsychotics have become the mainstay of treatment for mania and bipolar depression and for long-term prophylaxis. Quetiapine is effective in bipolar depression (an especially difficult condition to treat); however, it is often sedating and this will be a limiting factor for some. Others such as olanzapine are associated with weight gain. Most patients with bipolar disorder suffer from more, and longer, episodes of depression. Lamotrigine may be a useful drug for athletes in this situation. It is relatively non-sedating and well tolerated. In patients with psychosis or bipolar disorder particularly characterized by episodes of mania, aripiprazole might be a good option as it is non-sedating and has limited effect on weight. However, its side effect of motor restlessness (akathisia) and consequent impact on motor performance may be a problem. As with antidepressants there are no controlled data on the use of any of these treatments in sporting populations. See Table 10.2 for suggested treatments to consider in the various phases of bipolar disorder.

Lithium is an important treatment in long-term prophylaxis against bipolar episodes. Tremor is a side effect that may limit its use for some but it is an established and effective treatment that is safe if regularly monitored and if taken continuously. A careful dosing schedule is required as lithium has a narrow therapeutic window. If the dose is too low it is ineffective and it becomes dangerously toxic at just above the therapeutic dose. Continuous adherence is also necessary throughout treatment that can last for many years. It is not possible to phase out the drug for performance reasons, for example, during a period of heavy training or before an important competition, as this will precipitate an iatrogenic manic episode. There are no controlled trials of its use in athletes. A concern is that dehydration from sweating may lead to increased plasma levels, potentially into the toxic range and this is exacerbated by the possibility that strenuous exercise may decrease renal clearance. However, the concentration of lithium in sweat is higher than in plasma and in a study of four athletes taking lithium and running for 20 km in hot conditions it was observed that while they became dehydrated, lithium levels actually decreased. Lithium should not be ruled out as an option for athletes with bipolar disorder.

10.3.3 **Hypnotics and anxiolytics**

The drug class of first choice for anxiety disorders is the SSRIs, in preference to benzodiazepines that are sedative and likely to impair athletic performance.

138

Many athletes have problems with sleep from time to time, perhaps as a result of pre-event nerves, jet lag, staying in an unfamiliar environment, or competing late in the evening. As in non-athletes, it is preferable to manage insomnia using sleep hygiene techniques rather than medication. However, if medication is used the half-life of the drug is important. It takes four to five half-lives for a drug to be fully washed out. Nitrazepam has a half-life of 15–38 hours and thus is not a good choice. Not surprisingly, it impairs athletic performance the next day to a greater extent than temazepam (half-life of 8–22 hours). Zopiclone (half-life 5–6 hours) and zolpidem (half-life 2 hours) are better choices (see Table 10.2).

A non-benzodiazepine option worth consideration as a hypnotic is melatonin which has been shown to produce few hangover effects in athletes.

Case study 1

A 26-year-old rugby league player presented to his sports psychiatrist reporting an increasingly low mood with poor sleep, reduced enjoyment of activities, excess appetite described as 'comfort eating', and a negative effect on his relationship with his family. After a review that excluded excessive alcohol, thyroid problems, and other physical ailments he was consented to commence treatment with the antidepressant sertraline. This was chosen on the basis of evidence for its effectiveness and its side effect profile (low levels of both sedation and weight gain). There was a need to avoid side effects particularly during the playing season and he was commenced on 50 mg once daily which was titrated slowly every 2–3 weeks to a dose of 150 mg once daily with regular reviews in person and via telephone. Additional psychological approaches were used including cognitive behavioural therapy targeting symptoms of anxiety and anger. An improvement was noted at 3 weeks. At 8 weeks, symptoms had resolved with improved mood, performance, and family relationships.

Case study 2

Three months before the Olympic Games, a sprinter was diagnosed with severe depression and treatment with fluvoxamine was begun. Although this treated his depressive symptoms he noticed a sedative effect and without telling anyone he stopped his medication. Although successful at the Olympic Games his mood dipped significantly shortly afterwards and he performed poorly in a series of post-Olympic races. In the off-season he restarted fluvoxamine which again resolved his depression. However, he struggled to perform at his previous level over the following two seasons. With the support of his psychiatrist he learned to stop medication temporarily in the 2 weeks prior to important races and achieve a balance of mental well-being and elite performance.

Table 10.2 Possible 'sports-specific' treatment options	
Condition	Possible 'athlete-specific' treatments
Depression	Sertraline, agomelatine
Anxiety	Sertraline
Bipolar—mania	Aripiprazole, quetiapine
Bipolar—depression	Lamotrigine, quetiapine
Bipolar—prophylaxis	Lithium, aripiprazole, lamotrigine, quetiapine
Psychosis	Aripiprazole, quetiapine
Insomnia	Zopiclone, zolpidem, melatonin

10.4 **Monitoring the drug for the individual**

As in all other clinical situations, good quality treatment involves initial assessment, individualized follow-up, and regular review of the athlete by the prescriber. In the environment of a sports team there may be other medical and associated staff who can support this process.

10.4.1 **Initial assessment**

Prior to starting a psychotropic drug, baseline biochemical and physiological parameters should be measured (see Table 10.3).

10.4.2 **Follow-up**

The frequency and duration of follow-up can be agreed on an individual basis between the prescriber and athlete. It will be determined by the severity of the illness, the likelihood of adverse events or side effects, and practicalities such as travel, competitions, etc. The prescriber forms only part of the support team and others will be able to contribute to follow-up—perhaps reporting back corroborative information on any improvements or problems and undertaking further investigations. Practitioners should respect each other's expertise. A collaborative effort with clear task allocation will usually be in the athlete's best interests.

The benefits and risks of treatment are assessed and reassessed at each review and as regularly as practicable. The athlete's subjective view in addition to the prescriber's review of improvement will be equally important. Medication that is ineffective should be reviewed and likely discontinued. Quantifying and measuring sleep, appetite, and energy levels can be used to help assess progress. Validated measures such as the Patient Health

Table 10.3 Suggested investigations before prescribing psychotropic drugs		
Physiological measures	Weight	Some psychotropic drugs increase appetite
	Blood pressure	Postural hypotension with several drugs
	Body mass index	Monitor for metabolic syndrome (see Chapter 8)
Blood tests	Full blood count	To rule out anaemia or chronic inflammation or infection
	Urea and electrolytes	Low sodium with several drugs
	Calcium	To exclude hypocalcaemia as a contributory factor in mood disturbance and fatigue
	Liver function tests	Monitor for hepatic impairment
	Thyroid function tests	To rule out thyroid disease as cause of low mood, fatigue etc.
	Glucose	Monitor for metabolic syndrome (see Chapter 8)
Other tests	ECG	To check for QTc prolongation

Box 10.1 PHQ-9 patient depression questionnaire

Over the last 2 weeks, how often have you been bothered by any of the following problems? (Use '√' to indicate your answer)	Not at all	Several days	More than half the days	Nearly every day
1. Little interest or pleasure in doing things	0	1	2	3
2. Feeling down, depressed, or hopeless	0	1	2	3
3. Trouble falling or staying asleep, or sleeping too much	0	1	2	3
4. Feeling tired or having little energy	0	1	2	3
5. Poor appetite or overeating	0	1	2	3
6. Feeling bad about yourself—or that you are a failure or have let yourself or your family down	0	1	2	3
7. Trouble concentrating on things, such as reading the newspaper or watching television	0	1	2	3
8. Moving or speaking so slowly that other people could have noticed? Or the opposite—being so fidgety or restless that you have been moving around a lot more than usual	0	1	2	3
9. Thoughts that you would be better off dead or of hurting yourself in some way	0	1	2	3
Column totals		_____ + _____ + _____ + _____		
		= *Total Score* _____		

If you checked off **any** problems, how **difficult** have these problems made it for you to do your work, take care of things at home, or get along with other people?

Not difficult at all	Somewhat difficult	Very difficult	Extremely difficult
☐	☐	☐	☐

Reproduced from *Journal of General Internal Medicine*, 16(9), Kroenke K, The PHQ-9, p. 606–613, Copyright (2001) with permission from Springer.

Questionnaire (PHQ-9) depression scale can be used to supplement clinical judgement in monitoring the severity of depression and response to treatment (see Box 10.1). It can be used remotely (e.g. over the telephone) and may be convenient in athletes who are travelling frequently (the PHQ-9 is available to download at http://phqscreeners.com).

10.4.3 **Monitoring**

Physical health parameters should be monitored. Guidance is available on the biochemical and physiological tests required to monitor physical health (e.g. The Lester UK Cardiometabolic Health Resource). This describes the monitoring necessary when antipsychotic medication is prescribed and is especially focused on features of metabolic syndrome (see Chapter 8). Monitoring can be undertaken by the prescriber or delegated to another appropriate professional in the team (e.g. team doctor, physiotherapist, or strength and conditioning coach). Priority follow-up by a psychiatrist is recommended in cases where there is rapid weight gain (e.g. > 5 kg in < 3 months) or where there is the development of abnormal blood pressure, glucose, or lipids.

10.4.4 **Side effects and performance**

The effects of psychotropic medications on athletic performance are critical not just for reasons of safety but because an athlete who perceives a drop in performance may not want to continue that treatment even if there is an obvious clinical improvement. This applies to anyone who has sport as an important aspect of their life and not just to elite performers. However, there is lack of evidence on the effects that specific medications have on any aspect of performance and measuring a performance decrement is not straightforward. Running speeds may be slower because the quantity and quality of training has changed, perhaps as a consequence of the illness.

Elite sports teams have developed methods of monitoring and analysing athletic performance and these can used to monitor and adjust medication. For example, the Bradford Bulls Rugby League Football Club use a 'wellness app' to monitor well-being parameters such as sleep quantity and quality, subjective mood, fatigue, muscle soreness, and stress levels on a daily basis. These are correlated with physical performance parameters such as adductor squeeze, toes-touch flexibility, and ankle mobility tests to produce a thorough understanding and evaluation of the athlete's state of health. Importantly, it not only gives equal weight to both physical and mental health measures but sees the two as linked. The mobile app has been used to supplement standard clinical practice in monitoring a player's recovery from injury (both physical and mental) and progress through treatment.

10.5 **Prohibited drugs and Therapeutic Use Exemptions**

The World Anti-Doping Agency (WADA) produces a list of prohibited substances that is reviewed and updated annually. Most of the substances included in the list are, fortunately, not those that would normally be used in the treatment of mental health problems.

The drugs on the prohibited list that are directly relevant to psychiatric practice include the following:

- Modafinil, methylphenidate, and selegiline all appear in the 'stimulant' category. WADA also prohibits 'other substances with a similar chemical structure or similar biological effect(s)'. This may therefore include monoamine oxidase inhibitors such as phenelzine and tranylcypromine.

- Bupropion (along with caffeine and nicotine when part of a normal intake) is not banned but its use is being monitored. It is likely that if clearer evidence emerges of a performance enhancing effect from bupropion then it will join the prohibited list.
- Beta blockers which are occasionally used as an adjunct in the treatment of anxiety disorders are banned in some sports.

The principle to be followed is for the prescriber to check whether a drug they are considering is on the prohibited list and to do this in liaison with the club or team doctor (http://list.wada-ama.org). Care should also be taken as in some sports there are more specific regulations. For example, the International Archery Federation bans the use of any beta blockers both in and out of competition.

If medication is necessary but is on the prohibited list then a Therapeutic Use Exemption (TUE) can be sought to authorize its use. Updated details of the procedure can be found on the WADA website (http://www.wada-ama.org). It involves a robust medical assessment and a medical submission to the national governing body of that sport. In psychiatry, a potentially common situation is in the treatment of attention deficit hyperactivity disorder. Methylphenidate is a prohibited substance but can be used with a TUE whilst atomoxetine is not prohibited.

10.6 **Summary and conclusions**

The basic principle in using psychotropic medications for mental illnesses is to follow good clinical practice. This applies to athletes and non-athletes alike and in all cases treatment should be tailored to the individual. There is scant evidence on the effects of psychotropic drugs on athletic performance to guide treatment choice. Therefore it is necessary to apply sound knowledge of the pharmacology of each drug being considered and to use clinical common sense in making choices. The effects of medication need to be carefully monitored—both for effectiveness in treating the illness and for side effects. Additionally, in athletes, monitoring must pay attention to any effects on athletic performance. Finally, all prescribers need to aware of doping regulations and the use of TUEs and to be prepared to work alongside team doctors and sports governing bodies.

Further reading

Cipriani, A., Furukawa, T.A., Salanti, G., et al. (2009). Comparative efficacy and acceptability of 12 new-generation antidepressants: a multiple-treatments meta-analysis. *Lancet* 373:746–58.

Joint Formulary Committee (2014). *British National Formulary* (68th ed.). London: BMJ Group and Pharmaceutical Press.

Lester, H., Shiers, D.E., Rafi, I., Cooper, S.J., and Holt, R.I.G. (2012). *Positive Cardiometabolic Health Resource: An Intervention Framework for Patients with Psychosis on Antipsychotic Medication.* London: Royal College of Psychiatrists.

Reardon, C.L. and Factor, R.M. (2010). Sport psychiatry: a systematic review of diagnosis and medical treatment of mental illness in athletes. *Sports Med* 40:961–80.

Index

145